DR. SEBI'S TREATMENT BOOK

DR. SEBI TREATMENT FOR STDS, HERPES, HIV, DIABETES, LUPUS, HAIR LOSS, CANCER, KIDNEY STONES, AND OTHER DISEASES.

THE ULTIMATE GUIDE ON HOW TO DETOX THE LIVER AND CLEANSE YOUR BODY

Aniys Hendry

INTRODUCTION

D r. Sebi (Alfredo Darrington Bowman) was a natural therapist, herbalist, and biochemist. He is the founder of the USHA research institute, also known as the healing village.

Dr. Sebi employed the use of natural alkaline foods and herbs to cure various acute and chronic diseases. Doctor Sebi produced several medications and, in turn, used these medications to prevent and treat several diseases.

He ended up disappointed with Western scientific practices in treating his allergies, diabetes, and impotence. He went to see an herbalist in Mexico whom Bowman claimed healed him. After that, Bowman started his very private recuperation exercising in Honduras. He evolved a treatment that he called the "African Bio-Electric Cell Food Therapy," and claimed that it could remedy a wide variety of illnesses, inclusive of most cancers and AIDS, in addition to an expansion of continual conditions and intense ailments. He additionally advanced natural products. Bowman set up his center in the 80s near La Ceiba, Honduras, and marketed his natural products in the United States. He called his center the USHA Research Institute, placed inside the village of Usha. He began to make use of foods that are rich in alkaline to treat various ailments.

The diseases he cured are numerous. Examples are arthritis, lupus, cancer, diabetes, leukemia, AIDS, asthma, impotence, eczema, epilepsy, fibroids, heart disease, hypertension, inflammation, lupus, multiple sclerosis, sickle cell… and many others.

Those that he helped and were suffering from depressive illnesses obtained freedom from those illnesses and are living a healthy and happy life today.

Many dieters and alkaline food lovers are enjoying their health today because of the employment of Dr. Sebi's alkaline diets and herbs. They, therefore, declared that his diet had improved their well-being.

This African in Honduras grows to be recognized to have been married many times and had 17 children, his ideas on the origins of germs idea and factored in fake-Afrocentric claims about Africans' first-rate generic traits and their diaspora.

Sebi, who continued schooling and healing for more than 40 years, was at the center of numerous criminal complaints before his "mysterious death." During his early years, many claimed that the medical enterprise wanted to sideline him and his achievements.

CHAPTER 1: ABOUT DR. SEBI THE NATURAL HEALER

Doctor Sebi Alfredo Darrington Bowman was a natural healer, a herbalist who used different types of vegetables, fruits, and herbs to treat diseases. He was also recognized as a natural therapist and a biochemist.

Doctor Sebi was not a medical doctor; neither did he obtain a PhD. in any medical field. He was a self-trained herbalist, although he got loads of knowledge from his grandma. In his lifetime, he employed the use of several alkaline herbs and organic foods for the treatment of different types of illnesses. He did not use magic or charms to treat diseases, but he judiciously employed nature's gift.

Doctor Sebi intensively studied many vegetables, fruits, and herbs that are extremely rich in alkaline and use them to fight against diseases and miserable illnesses. During his thorough investigation of alkaline plants, he created a healing village named a research institute.

Dr. Sebi argued that the body gets sick when there is an accumulation or excess of mucus and toxins in the body. He said that we must first flush out all these substances for the body to get rid of diseases. The flushing out of these accumulated substances must be carried out using alkaline detoxifying foods and cleansing herbs.

Doctor Sebi was diagnosed with some illnesses before he became a herbalist. He suffered from impotence, diabetes, asthma, and obesity, which orthodox medicine could not solve. Seeking healing from his illnesses, he located a herbalist in Latin America who, with herbs, cured all these diseases successfully. Hence, he developed an interest in studying alkaline/electrically charged fruits, vegetables, and herbs to treat diseases.

The following are some of the diseases he cured with alkaline diets and herbs: different types of cancer, impotence, HIV, arthritis, lupus, fibroid, herpes, high blood pressure, sickle cell disease, diabetes, epilepsy, eczema, depression, hair loss… and many more.

Key Points About Dr. Sebi's Diet

There are essentials points you must consider before trying Dr. Sebi's diet. These points are described below:

- Doctor Sebi's diet consists of all the types of foods you desire except for animal's products.

- His foods are alkaline grains, alkaline vegetables, alkaline fruits, alkaline nuts, alkaline tea, alkaline seeds, natural sweeteners, and alkaline curative herbs.

- Doctor Sebi's diets are most effective in fighting different types of diseases. Hence, his diets prevent prophylactics and cure diseases.

- Doctor Sebi's diet can help sustain a healthy lifestyle.

- Dr. Sebi's diet helps in revitalizing, energizing, and rejuvenating the body.

- Dieters who truly inculcate the use of the Sebi diets testify that the diets have done great work in their bodies.

- He claimed that all infections grow properly in a mucus accumulated environment. He concluded that alkaline diets responsible for detoxification could help remove this mucus.

- Again, he believed that removing excess mucus in the body via detoxification would help you eliminate any disease in your body.

- Individuals who believe that good health is their utmost priority inculcate the habit of following the Sebi diets. They make you look clean and healthy.

How to Stick to Dr. Sebi's Diet

These facts are significant in following Dr. Sebi's diets:

- If you aspire to stick to the Sebi diet, take his diet 60 minutes before taking any conventional medicine.

- You must not use a microwave on your food as it makes it a slow food.

- Avoid the intake of canned foods.

- Follow all the food mentioned in his nutritional food lists.

- You must drink one gallon of alkaline water in a day.

- Avoid the intake of seedless fruits.

- You can follow all his diets simultaneously without any problems.

- You must not take any animal products while following the Sebi diet.

- Hybridized foods are exempted from his diet.

- The intake of alcohol is also exempted from his diet.

- Eat only the grains listed in Dr. Sebi's food list.

The Significance of Dr. Sebi's Diets

When acidic foods are reduced in your meals, it builds an environment that makes it easy to fight against diseases and prevent the invasion of foreign bodies. Hence, the significance of the Sebi diet is:

- The Sebian diet helps in the prevention and treatment of breast cancer.

- This diet facilitates weight loss due to natural vegetables, fruits, grains, and other organic foods.

- The Sebi diet has very low saturated fat, which also prevents and fights heart-related diseases.

- The Sebi diet has completely no cholesterol.

- The Sebi diet has no alcohol.

- The Sebi diet has no processed sugar.

- The Sebi diet boosts the immune system.

- The Sebi diet reduces the risk of contracting diseases.

- The Sebi diet prevents and combats diabetes.

- The Sebi diet prevents and treats strokes.

- The Sebi diet provides the body with the energy it requires.

- The Sebi diet helps brain function.

Dr. Sebi's Recommended Method for Combating Diseases

Dr. Sebi employed the process of cleansing and detoxification of the body, and he concluded that this method is a vital tool necessary in dealing with any form of illnesses in the body.

Detoxification of the body helps removes mucus stored in the body and helps remove surplus acidic materials, thus making the body free from disease-causing organisms. He employed the use of herbs that are essential in re-energizing and revitalizing the body.

Dr. Sebi's Nutritional Recommended Food Lists

Alkaline Grains List

- Fonio
- Tef
- Spelt
- Kamut
- Amaranth
- Wild Rice
- Quinoa
- Rye

Fruits List

- Peaches
- Plums
- Soursops
- Dates
- Prunes
- Bananas
- Cantaloupe
- Figs

- Prickly Pear

- Raisins

- Papayas

- Cherries

- Grapes

- Apples

- Mango

- Soft Jelly Coconuts

- Pears

- Berries

- Melons

- Currants

- Orange

- Limes

Spices and Seasonings

- Achiote

- Habanero

- Savory

- Oregano

- Basil

- Thyme

- Pure sea salt

- Powdered granulated seaweed
- Sage
- Tarragon
- Cloves
- Dill
- Bay Leaf
- Cayenne
- Sweet Basil
- Onion Powder

Herbs List

- Cayenne
- Dill
- Oregano
- Basil
- Onion powder
- Pure sea salt

Vegetables List

- Bell pepper
- Chayote
- Cucumber
- Wild arugula
- Avocado

- Green amaranth
- Dandelion greens
- Turnip greens
- Wakame
- Onions
- Arame
- Cherry and plum tomato
- Dulse
- Garbanzo beans
- Izote flower and leaf
- Olives
- Purslane verdolaga
- Squash
- Okra
- Tomatillo
- Kale
- Mushrooms except for shitake
- Hijiki
- Nopales
- Nori
- Zucchini
- Watercress

- Lettuce except for iceberg

Herbal Teas List

- Ginger
- Fennel
- Tila
- Chamomile
- Elderberry
- Burdock
- Red Raspberry

Alkaline Sugar Lists

- 100% Pure Agave Syrup from cactus
- Dried Date Sugar

CHAPTER 2: ALKALINE PLANT-BASED DIET

The Health Benefits of Alkaline Plant-Based Diet

If you are a vegetarian, vegan, or aiming to move in this direction, the alkaline diet is ideal. While all dietary plans can be built on a strong foundation of vegetables and fruits, a plant-based diet is an option for adhering to this way of eating. Not all vegan or plant-based diets are alkaline; many foods that are free of animal products can be processed and contain acidic ingredients, though once digested, many "acidic" fruits and vegetables become alkaline. One of the most beneficial, nutrient-rich foods for an alkaline diet is soy. Soybeans (edamame beans) are a great snack on their own, as is tofu, tempeh, miso, and other soy-based foods. When choosing soy products, look for organic, natural options, and avoid preservatives as much as possible.

Why Choose a Plant-Based Diet?

There are many reasons to change to a plant-based diet, from reducing meat in your diet overall, to implementing one or two "meat-free days" each week. If your current diet is very meat-heavy, this will take some significant adjustment, so it is best not to make the switch from red meats to full veganism overnight. Veganism or vegetarianism work best when whole, natural foods are chosen instead of packaged or processed options. A lot of marketing is involved in promoting meat-free packaged snacks and condiments. However, many of these may contain sugars, high amounts of sodium, artificial color, additives, and other unhealthy ingredients.

There is a lot of research to support a plant-based diet, and the high amount of alkaline in many fruits and vegetables means a good fit with the alkaline-based diet:

- The emphasis is on the whole, natural foods, which simplify shopping and selecting foods for your diet. This also makes meal preparation and planning more comfortable, as your focus will be on vegetarian-based eating, without meat as an option, and little or no dairy.

- A plant-based diet can help with weight loss, as vegetables and fruits are digested and used much more quickly than meat and dairy products. There are also fewer calories in vegetarian meals, even where the actual portion size is the same or similar to a regular meal, including meat.

- Meeting your goal weight is an outstanding achievement, and maintaining the weight is another task. This can be done more effectively with plant-based eating. There are not only restrictions on meat and dairy consumption, but on processed foods, which sometimes contain meat by-products (gelatin) and a high amount of preservatives, or artificial flavors.

- Soy is a major staple of a plant-based diet. The amount of calcium, protein, iron, and nutrients in soy products is comparable to meat and a fraction of the calories and fat. Soy is also relatively inexpensive and easy to find in most grocery stores. Tofu, tempeh, and edamame beans are popular ways to enjoy soy in almost any meal type.

- Enjoying a plant-based diet can reduce or eliminate food sensitivities to dairy and meat products, as these are no longer a part of the diet. Other food allergies or sensitivities may be less of a factor; once a more pH balance is established in your body, digestion becomes more comfortable, and health improves overall.

- It will improve heart health and cardiovascular function to prevent cancer, type 2 diabetes, and many other conditions.

Prevention is a big factor why choosing a plant-based diet, as many illnesses and diseases can be avoided in the first place.

The Benefit of Soy in an Alkaline Diet

When it comes to soy, many studies and findings result in positive outcomes and benefits of eating soy, of the dangers of increasing estrogen, and its impact on your health. Overall, soy is a healthy option for any diet, especially for plant-based vegan diets that avoid all meat products. For people with allergies to soy and soy-based products, some alternatives can be used to adhere to a vegan meal plan successfully. For most people, soy is a good option with the following advantages:

- **High in protein:** Soy can provide just as much, if not more, protein in your diet than meat. In combination with a balanced diet that includes fresh vegetables and fruits, your body will receive more than the required daily protein.

- **Low in cholesterol:** Plant-based foods are low in cholesterol, saturated, and trans fats, making them a good choice for good cardiovascular function and a way to prevent heart disease.

- **High in fiber:** Soy, like all vegetables and fruits, is very high in fiber. Not only will you meet your daily protein, calcium, and iron requirements by switching to soy from meat, you'll also receive a good dose of fiber with each serving, which increases metabolism and keeps weight at a healthy, manageable level.

- Vitamin B12 and other nutrients considered only available in meat and meat-related products are also found in some soy products. Fermented soy, such as miso and tempeh, contains a sufficient amount of B12 to meet dietary requirements.

- Vitamin D is often an ingredient in dairy milk due to being fortified, though this can be found in various soy products.

While only a small amount of this vitamin is required, it must be a part of your diet.

- Soy products come in many forms, textures, and flavors. Soft tofu varieties, for example, can be used to create puddings, cakes, and smoothies. Firm tofu and tempeh can be marinated and fried, baked, or sautéed with any combination of vegetables and ingredients. Soymilk is a great alternative to dairy and can be used with cereals, in smoothies, milkshakes, and as a refreshing beverage.

- **Easy to digest:** While some people have reported bloating and mild issues with digesting soy, in general, it's easy food for the body to digest and break down for nutrients.

Alternatives to Soy for a Plant-Based Diet

If soy-based foods are not an option for your plant-based diet, there are many alternatives to choose from. These foods contain high amounts of protein, calcium, and iron, which are found in meats and dairy products:

Coconut-Based Yogurt

Like dairy yogurt, vegan, coconut-based yogurt is made by cultivating a coconut bacterial culture from coconut to create a product with the same texture, nutrients, and a similar flavor to dairy yogurt.

Vegan Cheese

Most varieties of vegan cheese are soy-based, though a growing number of plant-based cheeses are made from vegetables and vegetable oils. The benefits of vegan cheese include a similar taste and texture to regular, dairy cheese. Vegetable-based cheese, as opposed to soy-based products, tends to melt easier, which makes this variety a preferred option for vegan grilled cheese and mac and cheese dishes.

Almond, Cashew, and Coconut Milk

There are many non-dairy milk alternatives available at nearly every grocery store and local restaurant. Almond milk is becoming nearly as popular as soymilk, as well as other nut-based kinds of milk, including cashew milk. Some varieties include a combination of almond and coconut milk, or cashew and almond, for a pleasant, nut-like taste that works well in recipes, smoothies, and cereals. More people are ditching dairy milk and cream for non-dairy options for their coffee and tea as well. Other alternatives include hemp and rice milk.

Nut Butters

Peanut, almond, and other nut kinds of butter are an excellent source of protein and energy. Just one or two spoons of these kinds of butter will provide a good boost of nutrients before a workout or an active day.

Other Soy Alternatives

Nuts and seeds can be added to stir fry dishes and salads instead of tofu and other soy foods to boost the protein and calcium content. Olive oil or coconut oil are both good alternatives for baking and cooking vegetarian dishes. Both oils have a neutral flavor that works well with any combination of ingredients.

Alkaline Fruits

Fruits are an excellent source of vitamins, fiber, energy, and natural sugars that can easily replace the need for sweet snacks and processed foods. When we shop for fruits, we tend to choose from a small circle or group of fruits that we are familiar with and comfortable with. The variety of limitations on what fruit we buy can depend on what's in season, how much of a budget we have to work with, and our cravings. Bananas, apples, oranges, and berries tend to be most popular, and for a good reason: they are delicious and easy to eat. Apples are best during autumn when they are in peak season and are available in many varieties of texture, taste, and appearance. During summer months, it's the perfect time to enjoy fresh fruits such as berries, bananas, and melons.

If you buy local, fresh fruits become less available during winter or colder seasons. Frozen fruits are another option to consider. They are just as healthy and more convenient, as they last longer and can be used at any time. Canned foods, even vegetables or fruits, should be avoided, as they contain extra sodium and sugar, along with other additives.

Which Fruits Are High in Alkaline?

All fruits have a significant amount of alkaline, which makes them all good choices for an alkaline diet. The amounts vary depending on which fruit and whether alkaline is either low, moderate, or high. Some fruits that contain acidic properties will convert to alkaline once digested, like tomatoes and citrus fruits, while others contain a high amount of alkaline before consumption:

- Blackberries, strawberries, and raspberries. Berries are a great choice in an alkaline diet due to their high amount of vitamin C and antioxidants.

- Nectarines, like peaches, are high in alkaline and make a great snack on their own or in a fruit salad.

- Watermelons are not only high in alkaline but also contain a good amount of potassium and fiber. They are an excellent choice for a snack and especially refreshing during the summer season when they are more readily available.

- Apples have a bigger amount of alkaline that's moderate to high, though they contribute a lot of nutrients that make them a preferred snack any time of the year. They can be enjoyed raw, stewed, or baked for a variety of dishes. Apples are also naturally sweet, which makes them ideal for desserts.

- Bananas are high in potassium, fiber, and pack a lot of energy into just one serving. One banana can provide up to 90 minutes of energy, an easy and quick snack before a workout, hike, or cycling.

- Cherries, similar to berries, are high in alkaline and fiber. They also promote regularity and a healthy metabolism.

Are there any fruits to avoid? With an alkaline diet, virtually all fruits are good options, making the diet an easy process to follow.

CHAPTER 3: HOW TO FOLLOW THE DIET

Rules to Follow

To follow Dr. Sebi's diet, you must strictly adhere to his rules present on his website. Here is a list of his guidelines below:

- Do not eat or drink any product or ingredient not mentioned in the approved list of the diet. It is not recommended and should never be consumed when following the diet.

- You have to drink almost one gallon (or more than three liters) of water every day. It is recommended to drink spring water.

- You have to take Dr. Sebi's mixtures or products one hour before consuming your medications.

- You can take any of Dr. Sebi's mixtures/products together without any worry.

- You need to follow the nutritional guidelines stringently and punctually take Dr. Sebi's mixtures/products daily.

- You are not allowed to consume any animal-based food or hybrid products.

- You are not allowed to consume alcohol or any kind of dairy product.

- You are not allowed to consume wheat, only natural growing grains, as listed in the nutritional guide.

- The grains mentioned in the nutritional guide can be available in different forms, like pasta and bread, in different health food stores. You can consume them.

- Do not use fruits from cans; also, seedless fruits are not recommended for consumption.

- You are not allowed to use a microwave to reheat your meals.

How to Prepare the Body

It should be clear that it is a restrictive diet low in calories. Many people believe that it cannot be used as a standard way to lose weight as it puts too stress on the body of a new dieter. Because it is low in calories and an intensive diet, weight loss can be seen, but the person needs to assess whether they can handle a low caloric diet. Being too ambitious with this diet might turn fatal, so if you want to try the diet, be careful!

This diet has been suggested to be followed throughout one's entire life, which might not be possible for a new dieter. With any diet, if you start cutting foods firmly and then revert to your old routine of eating unhealthy meals, the chances are that the weight loss and benefits you see will get reversed. This is a risk in this diet as well. When starting, set reasonable goals and don't go too strongly. Let your body get used to it and then start setting up more ambitious goals.

Drink Water

Smoothies are a drink, and by drinking them, you are ultimately fulfilling your water intake for the day. Dr. Sebi's diet requires you to drink one gallon of water daily, but that can be difficult. Dehydration is a serious problem that leads to anxiety. To prevent that, you need to drink lots of water, which the smoothie diet helps you with.

What You Should Not Eat

Foods that are not listed in the nutritional guide are not allowed to be consumed. Some examples of such foods are given below:

- Any canned product, be it fruits or vegetables, listed in the nutritional guide.

- Seedless fruits like grapes.

- Eggs are not permitted.

- No dairy product is allowed.

- Fish is not permitted.

- No poultry product is allowed.

- Red meat is strictly banned.

- Soy products, which are a replacement for meat, are also banned.

- Processed foods are not allowed.

- Restaurant foods and delivered foods are not to be consumed.

- Hybrid and fortified foods are not permitted.

- Wheat is not permitted.

- White sugar is strictly banned.

- Alcohol is banned.

- Yeast and its products are not allowed.

- Baking powder is not permitted.

Some other foods and ingredients have been cut off. You only need to follow the nutritional guide to know what you have to eat.

Alkaline Meal Plan

Among the diverse body parts, the liver is among one of the significant organs, for it has considerable capacity in body detoxification. Through this body detoxification, synthetics and other foreign substances like poisons and even defecation, pee, and sweat are expelled from the body. These substances originate from the unsafe meals that we eat like delivered foods, liquor drinks that we consume, cigarettes that we smoke, even drugs that we take for anti-infection treatment, and hormone elective drugs. These substances are the ones that our bodies attempt to take out every day.

When there are many harmful materials inside the body, the liver needs to keep up until its ability runs out. When our livers reach this point, vast amounts of poisons can be gathered in the body and cause many body issues and diseases. To anticipate this and keep up excellent health, we should go through detoxification diet and takes our liver into consideration.

A liver detoxification plan can be completed either on a three-day, seven-day, or twenty-one-day program. This depends on a firm focus on a diet with unprocessed and natural foods grown from the ground, entire grains, and water cure with enough measure of water or liquid other option. Nourishments that are wealthy in fat or sugar, caffeine, liquor drinks, unnatural and human-made nourishment, drugs, and low-quality nourishments would all be able to must be put to a stop, at any rate, seven days before the diet plan.

- **One to Three Days:** This is the period to start your fluid diet plan where you need to drink around ten to twelve glasses of water ordinarily alongside frequently squeazed lime juice. Even though it can indeed be challenging to execute this diet because of the weariness and slightness, light exercise can be included as a request to affix the method of flushing the poisons out of the body. Additionally, you should shun taking in any sort of milk or dairy item.

- **Four to Six Days:** Fresh organic products, vegetables, and entire grains can be expended like celery, apples, carrots, oranges, which would all be blended into one juice. The juice can incorporate your selection of leafy foods. Even though healthy nourishments are consumed, there are as yet liquid choices, for example, natural teas for a few cups every day. Suppers can incorporate cut vegetables like celery, carrots, broccoli, and spinach. Besides, you can likewise utilize soups that you can consume at regular intervals.

- **Seven Days:** Along with the leafy foods, the liquids are expended together. They would all be able to be arranged by having them crude or steamed. Additionally, you can consume rosemary tea and dandelion options, which can be useful for this period.

You can generally change the sorts of foods grown from the ground that you will use as long as you oblige the strategy. When you reach the seventh, you can participate in the typical diet, finally. However, there is still a restriction on liquor consumption for around one entire week after the detoxification diet. Most likely, this detoxification diet can have an enormous impact on the advancement and support of a healthy lifestyle.

Instructions to Detox Your Body with Alternative Therapies

Traditional Chinese Medicine (TCM) is a fantastic asset when figuring out how to detox your body, and is mainly prescribed for treating stomach related issues, for example, Irritable Bowel Syndrome; ceaseless skin conditions like dermatitis; weariness and despair; hormonal inbalances, for example, PMS; endometriosis and poor sperm count, and infertility (both male and female). It can create results with interminable conditions that Western methods neglect to help. At the point when joined with a detox diet, it can make clear improvements in a person's health and prosperity.

Self-prescribing treatment of ailments are not suggested; however, at some TCM focuses, you can talk about your side effects to the specialist behind the counter and get a suitable cure on the spot. TCM can be useful for treating individuals experiencing withdrawal from drug and liquor addictions. Liquor makes the liver and nerve bladder work irregularly.

Numerous drugs are processed through the liver, making it warmed and blocked, so the liver's blood gets frail and insufficient. TCM focus on clearing and supporting the liver and nerve bladder, while simultaneously treating the heart, to help quiet the brain and sensory system. Consolidating TCM and figuring out how to detox your body yourself is probably the best thing you can accomplish for your health.

CHAPTER 4: HOW TO NATURALLY REVERSE DIABETES AND LOWER YOUR BLOOD PRESSURE

Dr. Sebi's Nutrition That Cuts Out the Sugar

Taking out sugar might be more of a drastic action, but if there is any diabetic medical condition that requires this, then you are left with no other choice. However, don't lose hope, as there are still methods to cut out the sugar content of a food item without making the food item either bland or tasteless.

For your breakfast options, which include cereal, try to add dried berries, cinnamon, apricots, or other kinds of dried fruits, which will help give it a naturally sweet flavor that would be the best option for a diabetic patient. Another method that you can use to cut out the sugar content is to use strawberry or homemade raspberry sauce on pancakes and waffles rather than the sweetened syrup.

If it is possible, try to replace sugar with fruit purees as they contain natural sugars, and it is also one of the best options for a diabetic patient. This is most important when there are recipes that need you to use one or more cups of sugar for the ingredients.

When you want to prepare vegetable dishes, try to add some sweeter vegetables alongside strong-flavored vegetables. It will assist in sweetness and will be beneficial to the taste of the dish.

In that case, you will have to use a combination of ginger and carrots, mashed sweet potatoes with cinnamon, spinach with nutmeg, and other relevant combination which you find pleasing. When you buy pre-prepared food items, try to look for the food items that have the right labeling. This will also permit the diabetic patient to make the right decisions and buy the products that do not possess high sugar content. It is also possible to eliminate sugar if you try to cut it out little by little rather than all at once.

Dining Out For Diabetics

Aside from the everyday dose of insulin and a recommended workout routine, all the food a diabetic patient eats needs to be carefully prepared. All these attempts are to assist in controlling the blood sugar levels, and so it needs to be meticulous.

Going out to eat is no different from these rules, and you can do it happily with a little bit of effort when it comes to a diabetic patient.

There are several restaurants out there that offer healthy food options for customers who are not so healthy. These customers may include the likes of those who want to control their cholesterol level, their intake of calories, or people who want to eat healthy foods all the time.

It is not difficult to locate these restaurants that offer healthy foods for the different customers' needs. Locating fish, vegetables, baked or broiled goods, salads, and grain bread on a menu is easy, a majority of people choose these options. You should know that there are also restaurants that create their menus to show you the calorie and fat contents on their menus.

Meanwhile, some restaurants provide foods that are low in cholesterol, fat, and sodium and have a high amount of fiber. Low calories salad, low fat, or low-fat milk are mostly offered in different restaurants today. Some restaurants will also provide the customers with several options of preparation methods, which might include the healthier broiled style rather than the fried style, skinless chicken, and lean cuts of meat rather than the other popular, unhealthy styles which people like a lot.

Another drawing feature is that the majority of these restaurants do not place a bill for added changes in the menu contents or preparations, and they, in most cases, move out of their comfort zone to attend to customers who take care of their health by offering foods that match their health needs.

What Is High Blood Pressure?

If the walls of the arteries were to be clogged or packed with plaque, the blood flow would become restricted as it pumps from the heart to the aorta; when the arteries create pressure in a situation like this, the blood pressure becomes higher than it should be and this results into hypertension (high blood pressure).

Poor diet is the leading cause of high blood pressure in the United States as it has been reported that over 85 percent of recorded high blood pressure cases are rooted in a poor diet. More than any other race in the United States, African Americans reported more cases of high blood pressure. High blood pressure is a channel to other diseases such as kidney diseases, strokes, scarlet fever, enlarged heart, typhoid fever, coronary artery diseases, and tonsillitis. These diseases are rampant among African Americans who have a hypertensive health history.

High blood pressure is caused when the pressure of the blood flowing to the arteries is high due to the consumption of foods that are capable of clogging the artery walls. Blood is pumped by the heart to the aorta, then the arteries. Also, the walls of the arteries become narrow and hardened due to excessive plague caused by poor eating habits. The fact that as an individual gets older, the arteries get hardened bit by bit, and a bad diet will triple the possibility of high blood pressure is worthy of note.

How to Reduce Symptoms of High Blood Pressure?

Aside from clogged arteries, high blood pressure can also be caused by poor blood circulation. Synthetic drugs, processed foods, and unhealthy behavior patterns are also some of the numerous causes of high blood pressure.

These behavioral patterns include the following:

- Bad diet

- Tobacco intake

- Stress

- Excess of caffeine intake

- Fried and processed foods

- Overeating

- Aging

Symptoms of High Blood Pressure

According to Dr. Sebi, the high blood pressure symptoms can be likened to "navy seal snipers," as there are no signs that a person's blood pressure is high. The few noticeable pointers of high blood pressure have always been difficulty breathing, blurry vision, rapid pulses, and constant headaches.

Dr. Sebi's High Blood Pressure Diet

- Every high blood pressure drug in the market imitates water. This is why it is essential for you as an individual to drink a lot of clean water. To be effective, you will need to divide your weight by two and drink that much water daily. Why that much water? You may ask. Well, water thins the blood and so it is easier for the blood to pass through the arteries.

- Taking five different types of fruits (vegetables included) a day will prevent the arteries from getting clogged due to excess plaque deposits. Fruits and vegetables that contain a high percentage of antioxidants protect the artery walls from plague deposits. Such fruits include cabbage, tomatoes, oranges, seed grapes, and peaches.

- Foods that are rich in potassium help to reduce recurrent high blood pressure as it expels excess sodium from the body.

- Fiber containing fruits are also of high benefit to high blood pressure sufferers as it will lower the blood pressure while removing waste from the artery walls at the same time.

High Blood Pressure After Eating

Food-related high blood pressure knowledge is essential, as having no understanding of what foods to eat and to avoid is detrimental to the blood pressure level. No one wants to get high blood pressure from eating like everybody else. Here are some foods and habits to avoid

- Avoid overeating even the healthiest of foods.

- Avoid salty foods as much as possible as they transform into plaque in the artery walls. In essence, avoid sodas, baking soda, soy sauce, and meat tenderizers.

- Never eat canned foods.

- Eliminate things such as products high in sodium, dairy cheese, and alcohol from your diet.

- Do not eat in the evening.

- Avoid every other type of rice except wild and brown.

Dr. Sebi's High Blood Pressure Natural Herbs Medication

These herbs are highly recommended by Dr. Sebi as the ones that help to open the blood vessels, open the artery wall and eliminate the plaque that's built up inside it. These herbs contain natural alkaline and are high in minerals. These are not hearsays; they have been medically proved to be useful as blood pressure medication. These herbals are usually high in iron; some of these herbs include:

- Fennel

- Oregano

- Basil

- Yellow dock

- Cayenne

CHAPTER 5: THE 5 FOOD MUSTS

We've discussed the Dr. Sebi foods that you should make sure you have in your diet, so now we will look at the five things you must do when it comes to your food. That's a little ambiguous, but it will become clearer as you read on. These five things simply have to do with how you prepare or store y our foods, as well as things you should consume every day for a successful diet and a healthy body.

Cooking Your Food Is Not Going To Harm Its Electricity

For a long time, people have been spreading the lie that cooking your food will cause it to lose its electricity. A lot of people live their life thinking, "raw food is better than cooked food." According to Dr. Sebi, food can't be destroyed. You can eat it raw, you can eat it cooked, you can grind it into carbon and drink it, but it is still going to be electrical. If what you are eating is real food, you are not going to be able to destroy its energy.

You can't destroy any other energy, so why would you be able to destroy the energy in food? You can change its state, but you cannot destroy its energy. There are things that people call food but it's not real food. It is basically just garbage because it is full of starch. In an interview, Dr. Sebi talked about people who eat "raw foods" because it is "healthier." He said that when he first arrived in New York, there were many "raw" people, but they were eating raw starch, and they were anemic. They may have been eating "raw food," but it wasn't real, natural food.

You can eat food in any state that you want to because it cannot be destroyed. Food is energy, and energy cannot be destroyed. Just like Dr. Sebi has repeated time and time, why would his diet have been able to cure people of leukemia and AIDS if cooked foods lost their electricity?

Consume Plenty of Alkalizing Beverages Every Day, and It Doesn't Have to Be Just Water

You are supposed to drink a gallon of spring water every day, but you don't have to confine yourself to just plain spring water. You can get its alkalizing effects along with the benefits of other foods by mixing them into a delicious alkalizing beverage. One of the best things you can do for your body is to start every day with a glass of warm lime water.

As we all know, the body is made up of 60% water. Water helps to flush toxins out of the body, keeps you energized, and prevents dehydration. When you add lime, you are adding antioxidants. Limes are full of magnesium, calcium, vitamins A, B, C, and D, and potassium. Drinking lime water can help to promote healthier and younger-looking skin. The antioxidants found in the lime help to strengthen collagen, and the water will hydrate the skin. Lime water will also help your digestion. Limes work with your saliva to break down your food so that your stomach doesn't have as much work to do. This can help prevent constipation and acid reflux. Its vitamin C content can also help you out during the cold and flu season. The citric acid present in limes can also help to boost your metabolism, which will help you to store less fat and burn more calories.

Lime water isn't the only option you have. You can also enjoy any tea made from the approved herbs list. One of the most popular choices is ginger tea. Ginger is high in magnesium, vitamin C, and other minerals. Ginger tea can help to relieve nausea. It is a favorite among people who tend to suffer from motion sickness when traveling. A cup of ginger tea before you travel can help to prevent vomiting and nausea. If you are sick, drinking a cup of ginger tea at the first signs of nausea will help keep it at bay. Ginger tea is also able to help relieve congestion associated with a cold and allergies. Ginger tea is also able to improve your digestion. Drinking a cup of tea after you eat can help prevent bloating. It is also a great drink for people who have arthritis or other joint problems. Ginger tea can also help to relieve stress.

Keep Your Food Storage and Prep Healthy to Keep Your Food Healthy

Remember all of the Tupperware your mother collected over the years. Think about holiday gatherings with food wrapped in plastic wrap and those Styrofoam take-home containers from your favorite restaurant. While those may be convenient and affordable, they aren't conducive to a healthy lifestyle. Plastic has invaded our life in every way possible only because it is cheap, but what it does to our health and our environment is a high price to pay in the long run. Most Americans only recycle 14% of their plastic packaging, so most of this stuff ends up on our streets or landfills.

Anything your food touches has a chance to leech into your food, but this happens with plastic at a much higher rate than other materials. There are lots of different types of plastics, and substances get added to plastics to change how flexible it is, stabilize it, and shape it. BPA is one substance that gets added to plastic to make polycarbonate plastics. Phthalates are another substance that gets added to plastics to make them flexible and soft. Polycarbonate plastics are used in food storage containers, plastic plates, reusable water bottles, and even in the receipt you get at the store. Metal cans also contain BPA-based liners so that the foods inside aren't able to corrode the can. Paper cups are lined with BPA as well so that your coffee doesn't leak through as quickly. Most plastic containers will have a code on the bottom. If you see a number from 3 to 7, it could have BPA.

Phthalates are found in many different products and it can be harder to know if they are in certain items. They are in cosmetics, water, plastics, food, drugs, dust, and the air. Since 2008, manufacturers have removed some forms of phthalates from children's toys, and there are some countries that have banned them in packaging. The best way to avoid phthalates is to look for PVC or number 3. The Fair Packaging and Labeling Act requires manufacturers to mark phthalates, but it is not required when they are used in fragrances.

While the FDA considered BPA to be safe and that all plastics are tested and are supposed to be stable, it still has an effect on your health. Research has found that phthalates and BPA can mimic hormones, which can create an endocrine disruption. The endocrine system affects things from our sleep and immunity, to our reproduction and growth. Even BPA-free containers aren't free from these problems.

To make sure that your food stays healthy and doesn't soak up any of those bad chemicals present in plastic, it is important that you choose storage containers and prep items that are not made from plastic. Glass containers should be your best friend. Mason jars are a great option because they come in many different sizes, are inexpensive, and are reusable. You drink out of them, store salads, and soups, as well as seeds, nuts, spices, and herbs. Mason jars can also be used as lunch containers not to have to use plastic baggies.

There are also other glass storage containers out there if you don't want to store everything in mason jars. You can even find some that are made from tempered glass so that they aren't easily broken.

Stainless steel is also a good option. There are many different sizes and shapes, and you can find them in bento box-styles, insulated, and leak-proof. They tend to be more durable than glass containers, which is good if you have children. The important thing is to make sure that you buy 100% food-grade stainless steel and not aluminum. You will also want to make sure that your cutting board is not made from plastic as well.

You Should Make Your Veggie Stocks and Nut Milk

While everybody loves buying pre-made stocks and milk because of convenience, they may not be the best option for your health. When you purchase something pre-made, you have no idea what is in them. If you make them on your own, you will know what you are putting in them. When it comes to vegetable stock, the store-bought kind has a lot of salt in it, and it probably isn't pure sea salt. They probably used vegetables that aren't on the approved list as well. The great news is, making your vegetable stock isn't that hard. All you need is spring water, approved vegetables, and some spices. Allow them to boil together for some time, and you have vegetable stock. You'll also find that it tastes a lot better than the store-bought kind.

As far as nut milk goes, it's pretty hard to find one that fits the approved list. Almond and cashew are the most common. Get this; almond milk doesn't even contain real almonds. One industry insider has stated that a half-gallon of almond milk has less than a handful of almonds. Most of them also contain additives. A lot of vegan milk products contain carrageenan, which comes from seaweed and acts as a thickener. There is a lot of interest concerning carrageenan. Some say it is a carcinogen and others say that it can cause inflammation, ulceration, and contains no nutritional benefits. If you like using nut milk, and there are Dr. Sebi recipes that need walnut milk, you will need to make your own. Making your own nut milk isn't that hard to do, either.

Buy Your Products at the Farmer's Market When You Can

Shopping at a local farmers market gives you access to locally grown and fresh foods. The foods there are at the peak of the season, so they will be fresher and taste better. The produce hasn't traveled thousands of miles to get to you, either. It probably doesn't contain any wax coatings or sprays, either. You are also face-to-face with the farmer, which gives you a chance to ask them about the product and find out how it was grown. You may also find products at the farmers market that aren't available at your local grocery store, and the prices might be a little more reasonable.

CHAPTER 6: DISEASE REVERSAL WITH DETOXIFICATION AND CLEANSING

As the liver and digestive system are the main organs that deal with the toxins present in the body, to make them work efficiently, the detoxification and cleansing approaches are mandatory. The liver and digestive system are the main organs for the breaking down and removal of toxic compounds from the body.

How Does Detox Help Prevent Potential Diseases?

Human anatomy has been designed to live an exceptionally balanced life, but owing to our chaotic, sometimes out of control "modern world lifestyle," and its environment, our bodies and minds are subject to a constant influx of toxins. Our body functions are at considerable risk under this strain because they are sometimes weakened and may quickly cede to diseases and illnesses. A detox is like pressing a reset button on the body. This gives a break to our bodies and brains and slows down the digestive tract. Our bodies go into recovery mode after detox, so that we can concentrate on self-care and healing.

What Does Your Liver Do?

The liver is the largest organ of the body at about 1.4 kg and conducts a variety of essential functions, including:

- Helping produce the vitamin D required to make hormones.

- Removing toxic chemicals, microbes, and unwanted hormones from the body.

- Storing vitamins and minerals that including iron and vitamin B12 as well.

- Processesing the fats, proteins, and carbohydrates from the food you eat so you can get the energy and nutrients from whatever you consume.

- Creating products that are used by your immune system to protect your body from infections.

- Storing the sugar (glycogen) for future use when energy is required by your body.

Thus you can see, your liver, and your hormonal wellbeing, are incredibly essential to your overall health. If it doesn't perform well, you need to take the measures needed to help detoxify your liver and regain its healthy function. What you consume, drink, but even breathe and come in touch with through your skin, and then reaches your bloodstream, the body needs to process it. So maintaining a balanced lifestyle and adopting a healthy diet is incredibly essential to your well-being, especially your liver's health and well-being.

Symptoms of a Toxic Liver

Now the liver is metabolizing the hormones and other compounds through what is known as phase 1 and phase 2 pathways, two main stages.

If your blood is very toxic, it can have a detrimental impact on your liver's wellbeing, and you might be suffering from what's considered a congested liver. Symptoms of badly clogged liver include:

- Hormonal imbalance

- Weight gain

- Skin issues of rosacea, acne, dermatitis, rashes, psoriasis, and eczema

- Exhaustion

- Impaired digestion

- Chemical sensitivities

- Possible inflammation in the upper right portion of the abdomen where the liver is situated

Furthermore, you will increase your risk of dying from what is considered non-alcoholic fatty liver disease from an unhealthy diet and lifestyle, which is when you get too much fat in your liver. The fatty liver disorder is now America's most prevalent form of dreadful liver disease, affecting 70 million Americans — that's one in three people.

It may contribute to hepatic cancer, liver disease, and death at its worst. The warning factors for fatty liver disease now include:

- Type 2 diabetes and pre-diabetes

- Being overweight

- Possessing elevated amounts of fat in the body, such as cholesterol and triglycerides

- Recovering from other diseases, such as hepatitis C

- Exposure to contaminants

- Metabolic syndrome

- High blood pressure

Research has been conducted on 9,000 American people who have been followed for about 13 years. It showed a close correlation between consumption of cholesterol (from the diet they consume, including, for example, animal products such as eggs and meat) and hospitalization and mortality from liver cancer and cirrhosis.

That is how dietary cholesterol can oxidize, creating harmful and carcinogenic consequences. So consuming animal products is another way the liver will sustain damage, and that may lead to liver cirrhosis (liver scarring) and even hepatic cancer.

How To Detox For Digestive Issues

The Role Played by Toxins in Your Digestive Issues

Our lives are jammed full of more dangerous chemicals than ever. Our food, domestic cleaners, cosmetics, self-care products, and the air itself has environmental pollutants. Today only low-grade contaminants occur on most typically cultivated vegetables and fruits.

Healthy bodies detoxify all that may be dangerous. Yet over time, we're subjected to the contaminants and pollutants that are formed in our bodies and inflict harmful effects. The contaminants in your body will trigger your digestive system to quit functioning properly, resulting in gaining weight and a lot of other problems.

What Happens if the Digestive System Doesn't Operate Properly?

If your digestive tract is not operating well, contaminants overload the liver. Some contaminants can live long, which can make us feel ill and lethargic. The metabolism of the body slows down, and the accumulation of contaminants triggers fluid accumulation, bloating, and puffiness before you realize it. Some symptoms are:

- Gas/burping

- Sore skin

- Leaky intestine

- Heartburn

- Weight increase

- Bloating

- Stomach discomfort

- Persistent swelling

- Constipation

- Nausea

- Appetite loss

- Diarrhea and vomiting

- Extreme fatigue

- Mental distress

- Low-grade diseases

- Puffy eyes or bags around the eyes

- Allergies

How Toxins Lead to Digestive Problems

The more contaminants you encounter in your life, the more detrimental effects body parts face. Your food and environment decide how high your toxic load is over time, and then the toxicity triggers inflammation, which contributes to gaining weight.

How these toxins induce digestive problems is a complex procedure, which mainly happens in your liver, which is responsible for transforming contaminants into extremely reactive metabolites before these contaminants are fully excreted from the body. Although your body's liver is most damaged by toxins, the gallbladder, intestines, and pancreas are all important organs that retain toxins in your digestive system.

A healthy digestive system breaks down the diet to absorb the necessary vitamins and minerals that they can to expel the unusable products in your everyday bowel movements.

If the already mentioned symptoms linger, an unstable digestive tract is often correlated with:

- Allergies, mainly in food

- Hemorrhoids

- Obesity and weight gain

- Dehydration

- Nutrient deficiencies

- Diabetes

- Ulcers

- Small intestinal overgrowth

- Persistent diarrhea

- Signs of liver disease

- Skin issues like Psoriasis or Eczema

- Hemolytic uremic syndrome

- Brain and Heart problems

- Autoimmune conditions, like Multiple Sclerosis, Crohn's Disease, Celiac Disease, Lupus, Rheumatoid Arthritis, and more

How To Treat Issues Related To Digestive Tract Caused By Toxins

The best way to cure digestive issues induced by contaminants is to eliminate or reduce the intake and clear toxic accumulation from the body.

There are also different methods that you should seek to rid the body of contaminants before they induce stomach problems. Full body detoxification is also an effective remedy for toxin-induced digestive disorders, whereas other alternative approaches such as consuming the correct foods and utilizing supplements to enhance gastrointestinal wellbeing can help.

Your body, though, can only detoxify adequately with the correct food, lots of sleep, and good hygiene.

Paybacks of Detox for Digestive Issues

A digestive detox uses natural foods to wash away contaminants from the body. Digestive health is important to your wellbeing, so you can find advantages by cleansing up your body for your:

- Intestines

- Colon

- Liver

Detoxes can remove the body's toxic substances and pollutants before the pounds pile up. They improve your digestive wellbeing, too. Any contaminants within you will naturally grow removed before they have enough time to inflict damage.

A detox can help with loss of weight and support certain causes contributing to obesity, such as persistent inflammation. Specialists often consider that certain chronic diseases of proper digestive hygiene are easy to prevent.

People also feel more active following detox and have restored vigor. Since stress and contaminants impair the regular operation of the body, you might start feeling like your old self and bouncing back into good health.

Some Other Advantages of Detoxing For Digestion

Detoxing can also help clean the large intestine or liver, where the healthy bacteria breakdown the food. Furthermore, colon cleansing assists in other stomach disorders, such as constipation and abnormal bowel movements. So, it can also reduce the chances of colon cancer. Eating foods such as leafy greens and broccoli may help detoxify the colon, of course.

Digestive Problems and Detox Strategies

Be aware of what's going through your body when seeking treatment for stomach disorders that are perfect for your needs. For your digestive well-being, your dietary patterns, food nutrients, and detox remedies all play a role. For you, the right approach will also rely on your living style.

Many people consume more vegetables or nuts than products that are refined. Some use other foods to cleanse their bodies as laxatives. Natural remedies such as ginger or apple cider vinegar can help with negative symptoms. People use detox foods to remove contaminants from the body, varying from juice fasts to supplements or diuretics. Cleanses are also eligible for sale to disinfect either the entire body or a particular area, such as the colon.

CHAPTER 7: HOW DID DR. SEBI CURE CANCER?

D r. Sebi employed the use of alkaline foods and herbs for the cure of this disease. He stated that the body would remove any toxins present in it by simple detoxification and cleansing. He, therefore, engaged the use of electric foods that are also capable of revitalizing and energizing the body for adequate functions and activities. He also advised people living with cancer to desist from eating foods are not listed on his food list. Herbs responsible for the body's detoxification and cleansing will work best and remove all excess mucus present in the body that enables diseases to thrive. He generally detoxifies the various body organs such as the liver, gall bladder, lungs, prostate, breast, kidney, lymph glands... and so on. The detoxification process he employed is fully capable of removing every abnormal cell proliferating and spreading in the body.

Let us quickly look at the numbers of days and the herbs he used for detoxification.

Detoxify The Body With 14 Days Fast In Dr. Sebi's Way

The herbs listed below are the herbs used by Dr. Sebi for the detoxification and cleansing of the body from any toxic substances and mucus.

- Elderberry flower is used to detoxify the upper respiratory system, removing mucus from the body and lungs detoxification.

- Chaparral helps in detoxifying the lymphatic system and clears heavy metals from the blood and gall bladder.

- Eucalyptus helps in cleansing the skin while employed directly or consuming internally.

- Rhubard root helps in the detoxification of the digestive tract.

- Dandelion is a powerful plant that helps in the detoxification of the kidney and gall bladder.

- Mullein is used for the detoxification of the lung and helps in the activation of the lymph circulation in the chest and neck.

- Burdock root helps in detoxification of the liver and the lymphatic system.

- Cascara Sagrada helps in migrating stool through the bowels by causing muscle contractions in the intestine.

Hints on How to Get Positive Result

- Drink one gallon of water every day.

- You must not eat any food other than the ones prescribed by Dr. Sebi.

- Eat any fruit or vegetable of your choice from the food lists.

- Prepare any kind of meal as required from the food lists.

- Drink tamarind juice daily.

- Take Irish Sea moss every day

- Exercise daily.

- When you are done with the detoxification and cleansing process, you are not expected to go back to your formal habit of eating.

- Continue the intake of alkaline diets after completing your treatment because it will help you maintain your health.

How To Prepare The Herbs

1. The herbs should be bought from a reliable source, or you can collect them from a reliable garden.

2. Ensure you rinse off all dirt from them thoroughly.

3. Dry them by using direct sunlight.

4. Grind each herb separately to powder form.

5. Keep them in a dry and clean container.

6. Take one tsp. of each of the above plants and add three cups of alkaline water.

7. Allow them to boil for 10 minutes.

8. Take away the heat source and leave it for a few minutes to get cool.

9. Drain and drink.

10. Take one cup of the herb three times daily. This should be taken daily for 14 days.

Dr. Sebi didn't stop here; he continued the curing process of cancer using curative herbs that naturally energize and revitalize the body.

Cure Cancer With Dr. Sebi's Herbs

Let us look at the herbs he used to re-energize and revitalize the body for a perfect result. These herbs are listed below:

- **Anamu (Guinea Hen Weed):** Guinea Hen Weed is very effective in fighting cancer cells. The Anamu plant is used for the prevention and treatment of malignant cells and many other ailments, it also helps building the immune system, fighting pain, hindering the growth of tumors... and more.

- **Cannabidiol (CBD) oil with Tetrahydrocannabinol (THC):** Cannabidiol oil is employed for the treatment of cancer symptoms, which include pain, nausea and vomiting, lack of appetite, and difficulty with sleep. It can also be used to cure cancer. It contains many constituents such as anti-inflammatory, anti-emetic, analgesic, and appetite facilitating components.

- **Sarsaparilla Root:** This plant comprises an increased amount of iron that is significant for the treatment of cancer disease. It contains tumoricidal, taxifolin, astilbin properties. When this plant is taken, it is said to fight against hepatic carcinoma and melt the growth of tumors.

- **Pao Pereira:** Pao Pereira contains substances that remove the tumor and can also be employed for the prevention of cancer disease. The most interesting aspect of this plant is the ability to fight only cancer cells without attacking other cells compared to chemotherapy. Pao Pereira is a plant that fights against different types of cancer, such as breast cancer, ovarian cancer, brain cancer, pancreas cancer, and many more. It is a tree from the Amazon rain forest which caused a total reduction in the size of tumor cells and kill cancer cells.

- **Soursop:** Soursop is more effective than any other conventional form of cancer treatment, including chemotherapy. Several types of research has been carried out on this plant to observe its effect on a cancer cell.

- **Irish Sea Moss:** Irish Sea moss is very effective against cancer cells because it absorbs the substances that are toxic in the intestines and subsequently removes the cancerous cells via defecation.

CHAPTER 8: DR. SEBI'S RECOMMENDED LIFESTYLE CHANGES TO IMPROVE YOUR CANCER CARE

T he way and manner we live can have severe effects on our health and wellness. This also pertains to people who have been diagnosed with cancer. A healthy lifestyle can help in treating cancer and also assist you to be well. It might even make your long-term health much better.

Healthy living simply refers to adopting positive behavior alterations as part of a life-long and continual process. To select areas for your health improvement, we suggest you focus on these six factors, which we refer to as the "Mix of Six." Each of these factors helps the other and contributes to their effectiveness.

Accept Practical and Emotional Support

If you have a network of people who are encouraging you, it is advantageous for your health, mostly emotional encouragement or support. Research conducted has put side by side individuals who had the most and smallest amount of social support. It was recorded that those people who had the most social support had a much better quality of their healthy life, and they lived longer.

Below are some recommended ideas for building a support system:

- Request for assistance or for someone who can listen. Individuals, in most cases, want to assist but do not know how to go about it. Therefore, you will have to be precise and state your request.

- Enter into a support group. Sharing with other people who have related experiences might assist you to cope.

- Encourage others. This forms a healthy cycle of giving and receiving.

Manage Stress

Lowering your stress level can assist you in managing your physical and mental health. Below are some tips for managing stress:

- Make use of relaxation systems, which include meditation, yoga, and guided imagery.

- Make out short periods to meditate or think all through the day. This could mean taking time to be careful while washing your hands, chilling at a stoplight, or brushing your teeth.

- It can be of help put away 20 minutes or more each day for stress management practices.

Get Enough Sleep

Endeavor to sleep for 7-8 hours per night. This will help improve your health, mood, weight, memory, attention, control, coping ability, and so much more.

- Set a time for sleep and endeavor to follow it. Also, set weekday and weekend sleeping time the same way.

- Endeavor to make your bedroom as dark as you can.

- The bedroom temperature should be cool.

- Stay clear of screen time before sleeping. This means the time you set aside on smartphones, backlit tables, and TV.

- Do not take stimulants such as sugar, caffeine, and alcohol.

Exercise Regularly

Endeavor to exercise while cancer treatment is ongoing and after cancer treatment. This can assist in lessening weight gain, loss of strength, and weakness. Also, do not try to sit or stay on the bed for a long time.

These are Dr. Sebi's tips to keep in mind during cancer care:

- Build and form a fitness routine that is not dangerous for you.

- Add an aerobic activity. This will enable your heart pump.

- Also, add strength exercise.

- Look for means to walk when you should be sitting down.

- Cut short your sitting time by standing upright each hour.

- Join in short bursts of exercise all through your day.

- Integrate physical activity into time with friends, trips, and family events.

Endeavor to talk to your health care team about building an exercise plan that is secure and right for you.

Eat Well

A healthy diet can assist you to control cancer side effects, improve health, and recover speedily. It might also reduce your future chances of cancer. Below are some tips to assist you in building healthy eating habits:

- Add a collection of vegetables in each meal. The vegetables should be the majority of your meal, not an option.

- Consume foods that have high fiber. High fiber foods include beans, peas, seeds, nuts, whole grains, and lentils.

- Add prebiotic and probiotic foods to support a healthy gut. Probiotic foods are listed as sauerkraut, yogurt, kefir, or other fermented vegetables, including kombucha, kimchi, miso, pickles, and tempeh. While prebiotic foods have high fiber, they include Jerusalem artichoke, raw garlic, chicory root, dandelion greens, cooked or raw onion, raw leeks, legumes, beans, and raw jicama.

- Select lesser red meat such as lamb, goat, bison, pork, beef, and more poultry, fish, and plant-based proteins like beans.

- Do not consume processed meats like sandwich meats, sausages, bacon, salami, and hot dogs.

- Add monounsaturated fats and omega-3 in your daily diet. Good sources are listed as walnuts, canola and olive oil, olives, flaxseed, avocado, and chia seeds. Coldwater fish such as trout, salmon, tuna, and halibut, are good sources of the listed healthy fats.

- Consume lesser portion sizes. A simple way to begin is to use smaller bowls and plates when you eat.

- Study the period to know the time you feel hungry, and when you have eaten enough. In some cases, our bodies mistake hunger for thirst and otherwise. Endeavor to drink water first if you feel hungry when it is not food time yet.

- Do not take low-nutrient and high-calorie foods. These add up to fruit-flavored drinks, sweets, candy, and sodas. Select fruit or dark chocolate in lower portions as options to sweets.

- Consume less refined "white" foods. These are listed as white sugar, white rice, and white bread. These foods are produced and made in a manner that takes away minerals, fiber, and vitamins.

- Lessen the intake of alcohol. Men should endeavor not to drink more than two alcoholic drinks each day. Women should also endeavor not to drink more than one alcoholic beverage each day.

If you are taking cancer treatment, it is vital and necessary to work with a registered dietitian nutritionist specializing in oncology to build a safe eating arrangement for you.

Avoid Environmental Toxins

Reduce your exposure to environmental toxins that can raise your chances of having cancer and other deadly diseases, which include asbestos, formaldehyde, tobacco smoke, styrene (seen in Styrofoam), and tetrachloroethylene (perchloroethylene).

CHAPTER 9: ALKALINE DIET AND CANCER

C ancer cells themselves produce acid and increases the acidic content in the blood and the rest of the body. In this case, if a cancer patient continues to take foods that have a high level of acid, it is implied that there is going to be a big problem associated with the health of the individual.

There are many foods mentioned and used by Dr. Sebi for the treatment of cancer. He said that many herbs are very good for the prevention and cure of cancer. He claimed that many cancer patients do not need chemotherapy at all. All they need is to stick to the natural herbs that combat this illness.

Dr. Sebi also said that foods that are rich in alkaline contents are the best for fighting cancer cells. It makes the internal body organs to remain increased in alkaline.

More so, there is significant evidence in different studies that reducing the consumption of meat and the intake of vegetables, fruits, and some numbers of grains might prevent cancer. Well, this can not only prevent cancer, but it can also cure cancer if dieters can adhere strictly to the approach of Dr. Sebi's diet.

Many bodies in the U.S that investigate cancer stated that the patient's health is most likely related to his diet in such that when the patient consumes vitamins (vitamin C, vitamin A, and sometimes fiber), they might lessen the danger of cancer.

Also, the American Cancer Society mentioned that an individual who follows an alkaline diet and avoid foods that are processed such as high-fat foods, soft drinks, and junk food. Foods that are beneficial and good for the body are vegetables and fruits.

Dr. Sebi's Approach for the Cure of Cancer

Dr. Sebi employed the use of alkaline and electrically charged diet to attack cancer cells. His methods were not conventional at all; they are quite natural. In order to treat cancer naturally with the employment of Dr. Sebi's alkaline diets, there are so many factors that you must consider:

- The body must be in a state that is fit to fight against diseases.

- The body must be in an alkaline state.

- The acidic content in the body must be drastically reduced.

Consume living and raw vegetables and fruits

Ensure you drink one gallon of natural thermal or spring water every 24 hours. Although this water cannot be gotten in an ordinarily in the market wherever you get it, ensure it is 100 percent spring water.

- Shun the consumption of starchy and sugary foods.

- Ensure all your diets are alkaline.

Dr. Sebi's Detoxification Method

He used detoxification as his first approach in the cure of cancer. The major organ he detoxified was the colon, although he made the detoxification process to be 100 percent holistic, thereby detoxifying other organs such as:

- The liver

- The gall bladder

- The kidney

- The lymph nodes

He suggested that the body must be cleansed intracellularly to make the body free from infection.

He also energized the body by allowing it to invigorate and restructure itself with the consumption of enough quantity of sea moss plants.

The indications to detoxify are:

- Drink a lot of water.

- Drink a lot of tamarind juice.

- Fast for about 2 – 31 days. If you cannot fast, you can be taking vegetables and smoothies daily, and this will also help the detoxing of your body be effective. However, it is possible to do this for a longer period.

Remember that the herbs Dr. Sebi used to detoxify are Eucalyptus, Rhubard root, Dandelion, Mullein, Elderberry, Chaparral, Burdonck root, and Cascara Sagrada.

Dr. Sebi's Curative Methods

After the detoxification process, Dr. Sebi continued the treatment of cancer using herbs that subsequently rejuvenate the body and bring it back to a normal state. These herbs are:

- **Sarsaparilla Root:** contains a high amount of iron that is essential for healing cancer disease.

- **Anamu (Guinea Hen Weed):** it is very useful in fighting cancer cells.

- **Soursop:** this plant is better than chemotherapy at fighting against cancer. Several types of research have been carried on this plant to observe its effect on cancer cells. In one study, they looked at the effect of this plant on leukemia cells, and it was found out that it stopped the growth of these cells. The extract of this plant was also used in a breast cancer cell, and it was observed that the extract was able to diminish the size of the tumor, kill the cancer cells, and made the body immunocompetent.

- **Irish or sea moss:** this plant contains 91 to 103 of the minerals the body needs.

- **Pao Pereira:** the effectiveness of this plant is scientifically proven. It kills cancer cells of the prostate, ovary, brain, and pancreas. This herb is a great one. It is a tree from the Amazon rainforest and is employed as an alternative medication to treat above-listed cancer. During a research study, this plant's extract was applied to culture; the extract supports the normal cells' growth, killing the cancer cells. Not only that, but it also caused a total reduction in the size of tumor cells. This means it performs tumor-suppressing activities and can also be utilized for the prevention of cancer disease. This plant attacks only the cancer cells and doesn't attack regular cells as chemotherapy does.

- **Cannabidiol (CBD) oil with Tetrahydrocannabinol (THC):** can also be used to cure cancer. Dr. Sebi used this plant in his village, but in most cases, he does prefer other plants mentioned above.

CHAPTER 10: HOW DID DR. SEBI ADDRESS KIDNEY DISEASES?

B efore we consider any treatment, let us look at Dr. Sebi's fasting process, which helps in detoxifying and cleansing the body.

Dr. Sebi said, "Detoxification is at the heart of getting rid of kidney problems associated with mucus out of the body; there are no other ways that will bring the required result." Therefore, fasting is an essential factor that can help detoxify the body, especially the kidney. Fasting helps your body, including the blood, kidney, and liver, to experience cleansing and detoxification. For you to achieve a cure for kidney problems, you have to be willing to make a sacrifice like the one you are about to undergo.

Detoxifying your body could end with your kidney problems, depending on how serious you engage in the methods because they are not easy to eliminate out of the body.

The herbs used for fasting to detoxify the kidney are:

- Sea moss plant
- Linden leaf
- Nopal plant
- Elderberry

- Burdock root

- Stinging nettle root

When you collect this plant, ensure you rinse them thoroughly with running tap water. You can dry them through direct sunlight.

These should be taken in the morning and before going to bed for 30 days.

There are many other fruits and vegetables that are approved by Dr. Sebi you can take during this process. These fruits and vegetables include watermelon, berries, mushroom, zucchini, cactus plants, and leafy green. You can also take tamarind juice and water.

You are not required to take any solid foods even if listed in the food lists within these 15 days of detoxification. Foods such as seeds, grains, and nuts are not accepted. You can consume these after the curing process has ended.

Some of Dr. Sebi's products used for cleansing and detoxification are Bio-Ferro, Viento, and Chelation. You can buy them in drsebiscellfood.com.

If you cannot afford the already prepared product, you can buy the detoxifying and cleansing herbs discussed above.

Cure Kidney Problems in Dr. Sebi's Way

Dr. Sebi, in one of his lectures, spoke extensively on how he handled kidney problems, especially acute and chronic kidney diseases.

This process should begin immediately after the fasting process has ended.

First, use iron liquid, which replenishes the number of minerals needed for the body.

Dr. Sebi's liquid Iron Plus and Bio Ferro provide an increased amount of iron to purify the blood and remove all toxic substances in it. The Bio Ferro helps in increasing the frequency of urination to assist in toxin elimination.

Second, employ alkaline herbs, which contain a big amount of potassium. This helps the kidney to ensure easy urination.

The Dr. Sebi potassium phosphate, known as FOCUS, is a natural diuretic that helps in flushing out excess fluid, toxins, and acids in the body. This herb contains an increasing amount of magnesium, calcium, and phosphates.

Ensure you follow the Dr. Sebi instructions written on the package and continue to take the herbs until you achieve your desired result.

Treatment and Passing of Kidney Stones

The treatment of kidney stones requires the intake of alkaline herbs that are beneficial for consumption as food and as medicinal herbs. This means you have to consider both methods to be able to fight kidney abnormalities and problems.

The diet, which comprises vegetables, fruits, and grains, contains high amounts of magnesium and calcium because a reduced amount of these minerals could result in kidney stones problems.

Let us look at the herbs that are effective for the treatment and ejection of kidney stones.

Herbs Used for the Treatment and Ejection of Kidney Stones

Some herbs are very effective for fighting kidney stone disease. Some of these herbs are very common and will help you greatly to cure kidney stones and its ejection.

The herbs perform their functions by relieving edema in the ureter mucosa, decreasing spasms that occur as a result of irritation caused by kidney stones, and improving the flow of urine.

Examples of these herbs are:

- Saw palmetto fruit

- Dandelion leaf

- Lobelia flower, seed, and leaf

- Goldenrod leaf or flower

- Horsetail leaf

- Khella seed

- Madder root

- Gravel root

- Horse chestnut fruit

- Corn silk

- Couch grass

- Hydrangea root

Constituents and Scientific Backup of Kidney Stone Removal Herbs

Saw Palmetto Fruit

Saw palmetto fruit contains many ethyl esters of fatty acids, enzymes, tannins, resins, terpenoids, and sitosterols.

It is a reliable plant used for the treatment of Benign Prostate Hyperplasia (BPH). The herb contains tonic that helps the urinary tract, and it is used for both male and female sufferers.

This fruit contains spasmolytic effects, making it easy for the removal of stones, and it also benefits patients with dysuria and tenesmus. This herb reduces the pressure on the bladder and has a sedative effect on an irritated detrusor, which assists sufferers with bladder and prostate abnormalities.

Dandelion Leaf

This plant leaf is a very effective leaf which helps in the tonification and detoxification of the liver and kidney. The leaf is a strong diuretic, and it is compared to furosemide in animal studies. It has also been carried out in humans, and it was discovered that the effects are similar. Animal studies have shown that dandelion leaf is important in the removal of kidney stones via the direct passage.

Dandelion is one of the major sources of potassium with about 4.25% potassium compared to other drugs, which contain a lesser amount. It can be used as a diet and medication because of its ability to improve the urinary, biliary system.

Lobelia Flower, Seed, and Leaf

Lobelia contains powerful relaxant and antispasmodic effects that assist the urinary stones to pass through the ureters easily. This plant is regarded as acetylcholine antagonists though other mechanisms may speak for its broncho and ureter-relaxing effects.

Goldenrod Leaf or Flower

This herb is used as a strong urinary stimulant, which help improve of diuresis and reduce albuminuria in the kidney.

It is also very important for the treatment of nephritis and helps stabilize the body immediately after the kidney has discharged the stones. This means it should be used immediately after the kidney stone has been ejected.

The presence of flavonoids in the plant helps repair the kidney, blood vessels, and connective tissues surrounding the kidney.

Horsetail Leaf

Horsetail leaf is very effective to repair of connective tissues that surrounds the kidney and the lungs due to the presence of silica component in it.

Horsetail also helps in diuresis, and it is a general metabolic stimulant that increases connective tissue resistance. It is important in both acute and chronic removal of kidney stones.

Khella Seed

Khella plant, especially the seed, contains khellin and visnadin as its active components, which make it useful by acting as a mild calcium–channel blocker in the dilation of the ureters.

Visnadin contains some smooth-muscle relaxing components which is associated with the non-standard calcium-channel activity.

The active components present in Khella seed are excellently absorbed and have reduced toxicity as evidenced by the almost total lack of side effects with long-term use in the treatment of an individual with asthma.

Corn Silk

Corn silk is a very important herb as it is used for increasing the easy flow of urine, and it contains a demulcent property that helps in reducing irritation from stones and facilitating its easy removal.

This plant should be collected fresh, especially when it is still very green, in order to prevent the consumption of a low-quality herb.

Madder Root

Madder root is significant and used by patients with kidney problems because it has a spasmolytic effect on the ureters and enables the free passaing of stones. This plant was studied, and it has been proved to contain calcium-channel antagonizing effects, which might contribute to relaxing the muscles.

This plant is also used to prevent calcium and phosphate oxalate salts from forming kidney stones in the body.

Gravel Root

This plant used for the treatment of urinary tract.

Gravel root can dissolve concretions. It is used for the treatment of urethritis, cystitis, irritable bladder, and fluid retention.

Horse Chestnut Fruit

This plant is used to treat various health conditions because of the presence of anti-edema properties known as escin. Escin reduces small pore number and diameter in capillary endothelium, thereby decreasing fluid seepage into the tissues (Longiave D. et al. 1978).

The presence of calculi in the ureter is easily removed with the use of this plant. The plant has anti-edema properties that help in the production of enlargement of the internal diameter of the ureter, thereby helping the stones to migrate easily even in resistant cases.

Couch Grass

This plant is a saponin and mannitol-containing diuretic that contain some silica. This herb helps in the repair of irritated mucous walls and has been used to treat prostatic adenoma.

This plant helps in the easy removal of stones and helps in repairing and preventing the recurrence of kidney stones.

Hydrangea Root

This plant is important and useful for the easy removal of stones. It is also helpful for sufferers who have urinary tract infections and prostate enlargement.

CHAPTER 11: ALKALIZING FOODS THAT CLEANSE THE LIVER

Every day, our liver works incredibly hard to shield us from the harmful effects of metabolic acid, and it is possible for our liver to get exhausted, which greatly affects our wellbeing.

There are seven foods that will help you clean your liver naturally involve regular. The main way the body transfers digestion, diet, and environmental acid is through the liver to detoxify and purify the bloodstream through constantly cleansing the blood of toxins via the gastrointestinal tract, the skin, and the respiratory system. Yet your whole body may be thrown out of control and your wellbeing seriously impaired when your liver is overworked owing to pain or prolonged access to acid.

As the liver is also responsible for alkalizing bile development, detox is also metabolically essential for physiological, environmental and dietary acid break-down and removal of your lifestyle. It is incredibly essential to alkalize the liver with an alkaline lifestyle and diet. Without a well-functioning liver, the body cannot cleanse and disinfect metabolic and dietary acid, which is a nutritional catastrophe receiver.

Therefore, you may want to start adding seven essential alkalizing foods into your diet to preserve a stable alkaline liver.

Garlic and Onion

Garlic produces a variety of sulfur-containing compounds essential for the nutrition and digestion of the body. This bulbous onion relative also includes allicin and selenium, two important nutrients that have been shown to shield the liver from acidic damage and enable it to detoxify.

Grapefruit

Grapefruit has two effective liver cleansers, it's high in natural vitamin C and antioxidants. Grapefruit produces compounds that balance excess acids, including garlic. This also includes a flavonoid compound named naringenin, which allows acids to bind and be absorbed in the liver and not to be retained in the fatty tissues.

Green Grasses

Green grasses are filled with chlorophyll, the key molecule of green grass which buffers excess of metabolic and dietary acids, including wheat and barley grass. Chlorophyll production from green grasses also helps detoxify the small intestines and liver and maintain the body alkalinized.

Green Vegetables

Leafy, gourd, arugula, dandelion leaves, spinach, mustard greens, and chicory also produce various purification compounds that neutralize heavy metals that can heavily bear on the liver. Leafy greens often remove from the body pesticides and herbicides and facilitate the formation and distribution of alkaline bile cleansing.

Avocado

Rich in glutathione-producing compounds, avocados vigorously foster liver safety and improve the healing forces against toxic acid overload. Many studies have shown that consuming 1 or 2 avocados a week will heal a weakened liver in as little as 30 days.

Dr. Robert O. Young tells his patients to consume an avocado every day.

Walnuts

Walnuts, which include high l-arginine, amino acid, glutathione, and omega-3 fatty acids, also lead to the detoxification of the liver from disease-induced ammonia. Walnuts often help absorb oxygen, and extracts from their shells are also used in liver purification formulae.

Tumeric

Turmeric, one of the most effective foods for healthy liver maintenance, has proven that it effectively defends the liver from oxidative damage and also regenerates weakened liver cells. Turmeric also stimulates natural bile development, decreases engorged hepatic ducts, and increases the overall function of the gallbladder, another organ that purifies the blood.

CHAPTER 12: DEALING WITH HERPES

D r. Sebi developed five effective herbal products that have helped a lot of people to heal herpes. These natural products are what you need to cure herpes.

Below are the main ingredients contained in Dr. Sebi's products for herpes:

- AHP Zinc Powder

- Triphala

- Pure extract giloy tablets

- Punarnavadi Mandoor

- AHP Silver Powder

Let us do a detailed analysis of the elements contained in these products.

AHP Zinc Powder

The term AHP stands for ayurvedically herbo purified. The purification of zinc is done with decoctions of natural herbs such as Aloe Vera to produce AHP zinc powder. AHP zinc power is of a better benefit than the usual zinc tablets you consume. AHP zinc powder is prepared from naturally occurring zinc, making it very easy for your body to absorb.

AHP zinc powder also has the main qualities of some of the herbs used in preparing it. Modern medicine also acknowledges the importance of zinc for herpes treatment, but it is better to use AHP zinc powder instead of zinc tablets. AHP zinc powder is safer and more effective in treating herpes.

Triphala

Triphala contains three outstanding herbal combinations. The three herbs that make up Triphala are harad, amla, baheda.

These three herbs have not only been acknowledged for their potency by Dr. Sebi, but other medical experts have conducted research on these three great herbs and praised its efficacy.

This herbal combination is a good one that can be taken by both healthy people and people infected with the herpes virus.

This herbal combination can clean the unwanted materials and toxins in your body and help purify your blood and many organs in your body.

Dr. Sebi didn't only administer this herbal combination to his patients, but he also took it daily for optimal health and longevity.

Pure Extract Giloy Tablets

Pure Extract Giloy tablets are produced manually from the extracts of the best quality Giloy.

Giloy is the perfect herb to improve your immunity and fight sexually transmitted diseases (STDs)

Dr. Sebi himself was a big fan of Giloy, and now, modern medical experts have accepted that Giloy can help your body fight off many diseases and improve health.

Punarnavadi Mandoor

Punarnavadi mandoor is not a herbs purified mineral, but a healthy herbomineral created from the combination of herbs and mineral. Punarnavadi mandoor is an extraordinary combination of healthy minerals such as calcium, iron, and great herbs such as shunti, punarnava, alma, etc. This herbomineral combination works perfectly on the liver and helps to eliminate toxins in the liver.

Dr. Sebi administered this herbomineral combination to many of his patients, and the reason for this is that the liver's function was disrupted during infection, and Punarnavadi Mandoor is the perfect option to bring the liver function back to normal.

AHP Silver Powder

Ayurvedically herbo purified (AHP) is a process that involves purifying various minerals in herbal decoctions, making them useful for medication,

AHP ensures that the minerals maintain their excellent abilities and absorb the nutrition and qualities from the herbs, which they are purified into.

AHP powder is exceptionally helpful to your health, especially your nervous system. Dr. Sebi administered AHP Silver Powder to several of his patients with herpes, and the results were always good.

What makes AHP Silver Powder effective for herpes is that it works on your neurons, the very place where the herpes virus in your body use as their home and hiding place.

AHP Silver Powder works by sending silver nanoparticles into your neurons to eliminate and flush out the herpes virus in your neurons.

Curing Herpes With Dr. Debi Diet on a Budget

Dr. Sebi's way of curing herpes is a simple process, and that is to nourish and detoxify the body. With this process, if you are looking to get rid of herpes on your body on a budget, here are some of the things you need to do:

Herbs and Fasting

One of the first things you can do is fast during the detoxification period, where you are taking in the necessary herbs alongside iron. On many occasions, Dr. Sebi has highlighted the importance of iron when healing. This means that during this period, we can use the combination of green juices, water, and herbs for proper detoxification.

Herbs and the Alkaline Diet

Following the alkaline diet while following the herpes healing process is important. The alkaline diet is one where you consume vegetables and other essential meals with the restriction of meat and other starchy meals.

The ingestion of starch and meat is something Dr. Sebi has stressed as something we need to avoid when healing herpes. We also have a recipe list that you can follow to help you stay on the alkaline diet while curing your herpes.

This means that your body is cleansed of whatever might be fighting the healing process while you replenish the body and boost your immune system.

Overall Guide

- At this point, you would avoid cooked food as much as possible.

- You would also take out any acid-forming foods from your diet.

- Fast while you take water and herbs.

- Once you have completed your fast, you would need to take fruits and vegetables to improve the healing process.

- Once your herpes is gone, you would need to continue with the Dr. Sebi recipes for a while to keep you healthy and make the healing process a permanent one.

Herpes is curable, as we know, with all we have learned from Dr. Sebi, and it can be done on a budget as well. You do not need to spend a fortune to get this done, and all you have to do is follow the simple process highlighted here.

Dr. Sebi's Herbs for Curing Herpes

For Dr. Sebi's herbs for herpes to work effectively for you, you have to start with the cleansing herbs.

Below are some of the cleansing herbs you need to take:

Cleansing Herbs

- **Mullein:** Mullein helps to cleanse the lung and also helps to activate lymph circulation in your neck and chest.

- **Sarsaparilla root:** Sarsaparilla root helps to purify the blood and target herpes. Jamaican sarsaparilla roots are highly recommended because it is a great source of iron, and it is good for healing. This herb contains smitilbin, phenolic compounds, triterpenes, sarsaparilloside, and parillin. It is a therapeutic herb that helps in detoxification and blood purification. This herb is also effective against genital herpes, code sores, dermatitis, shingles, and autoimmune problems. It is also important for the treatment of cancer, especially breast cancer.

- **Dandelion:** Dandelion helps to cleanse the gallbladder and the kidney. Dandelion is rich in iron and potassium. It is one of the common herbs that are important for the curing of different diseases. It helps with cleansing and detoxification of toxic substances in the body. Dandelion is used for the treatment of herpes, hypertension, HIV/AIDS, urinary tract infection, breast cancer, skin infection, and hypoglycemia

- **Chaparral:** Chaparral helps to cleanse harmful heavy metals from your gallbladder and blood and also cleanse the lymphatic system.

- **Eucalyptus:** You can use Eucalyptus to cleanse your skin through sauna or steam.

- **Guaco Herb:** Guaco heals wounds, cleanses the blood, promotes perspiration, increases urination, keeps your respiratory system healthy, and improves digestion. Guaco plant is an anti-septic, operative, anti-bacterial, tonic, depurative, hemostat, fungicide, cholagogue, febrifuge, and laxative. This plant contains a high content of iron, strengthening the immune system, and also contains potassium phosphate that makes it effective against the herpes virus. It is also a fever reducer, and helps in removing defective mucus in the body.

- **Cilantro:** Cilantro helps to remove heavy and harmful metals from your cells, and this is essential to heal herpes because the herpes virus hides behind your cell walls.

- **Burdock root:** Burdock root helps to cleanse the lymphatic system and the liver.

- **Elderberry:** Elderberry helps to remove mucus from the lungs and upper respiratory system.

Revitalizing herbs are what can heal the herpes virus. Revitalizing herbs are herbs and oils that target the herpes virus specifically. It is important you take these revitalizing herbs after cleansing and detoxifying your body so that the herbs can completely clean your body.

Here are the Dr. Sebi's herbs that can heal the herpes virus:

- **Pao Pereira:** Pao Pereira effectively helps to subdue the herpes virus, and it also inhibits the duplication of the herpes virus genome. This herb is an awesome herb to help to fight the herpes virus.

- **Pau d'Arco:** The chemical constituents contained in Pau d'Arco have shown in vitro anti-viral properties against HSV-1 and HSV-2, and other viruses such as poliovirus, influenza, and vesicular stomatitis virus.

- **Oregano Essential Oil:** Oregano essential oil is a great anti-viral that can suppress the herpes virus. It works best at ninety percent concentration. Apply essential oregano oil to your lower spine because your lower spine is the point where HSV-2 is dormant. You can also apply it to your genital area and under your tongue.

- **Ginger Essential Oil:** Ginger essential oil can kill the herpes virus on contact. But you should dilute the ginger essential oil with a carrier oil The ginger essential oil has the same effect as the oregano essential oil.

- **Sea Salt Bath:** Sea salt helps to absorb electrolysis through your skin during a herpes virus outbreak. To succeed, you need to add a cup or half a cup of sea salt into a tub filled with warm water and soak your skin in it for some time. Ensure that the sea salt dissolves completely.

- **Holy Basil:** Stress is one of factors that can trigger a herpes outbreak through adrenal fatigue. Holy basil is an adaptogen that relieves adrenal fatigue and prevents the outbreak of herpes through stress.

- **Conconsan Plant:** This plant is an African plant. The highest concentration of potassium phosphate is embedded in it, which fights against the herpes virus.

- **Purslane:** This plant is grown yearly in cold climate. It grows up to about 45cm. It is loaded with a rich amount of iron components. It is reported that this plant is effective for the treatment of herpes simplex virus.

- **Kale:** Kale is a rich source of calcium, antioxidants, and anti-inflammatory components. It is also loaded with more lysine. Lysine is an amino acid that is essential in suppressing the herpes virus. Lysine helps to prevent the multiplication of the herpes simplex virus.

- **Blue Vervain:** This herb is therapeutic. It contains a vast amount of iron and helps in combating herpes simplex virus.

- **Lams Quarters (Pigweed and Wild Spinach):** This plant is rich in iron, and it helps in boosting the immune system.

- **Yellow Dock:** Yellow dock contains a rich amount of iron, and it is a tonic. It is important for the treatment of different diseases such as sexually transmitted diseases, intestinal infections, arthritis, and more. It contains Lysine, which hinders the multiplication and growth of viral cells in the body.

How to Extract Essential Oils for Herpes

There are numerous oils for herpes, and the one thing that we have to consider is the extraction process. The proper extraction of these oils from their natural sources is a delicate process that requires a lot of experience and the right materials. There are numerous methods of extracting essential oils, but we are going to cover the two most important techniques, which are steam distillation and cold pressing.

Steam Distillation

The process of steam distillation makes use of steam and pressure for the extraction process. This process is a simple one, but without the right expertise, it can go wrong. The raw materials are placed inside a cooking chamber made of stainless steel, and when the material is steamed, it is broken down, removing the volatile materials behind. When the steam is freed from the plant, it moves up the chamber in gaseous form through the connecting pipe, which goes into the condenser.

Once the condenser is cool, the gas goes back into liquid form, and this is the essential oil that can be collected from the surface of the water.

Cold Pressing

The cold pressing process extracts oils from the citrus' rind, and the seed's oil. This process requires heat but not as much heat as the steam distillation process with a maximum temperature of 120F for the process to go as planned.

The heated material is placed in a container where it is punctured by a device that rotates with thorns. Once puncturing is complete, the essential oils are released into a container below the puncturing region. These machines then make use of centrifugal force to separate the essential oil from the juice.

Both processes are essential, and it has to be done properly with the right level of information from experts who know a lot about the process, if not a lot more harm than good can and will be done.

CHAPTER 13: HOW TO CURE HIV USING DOCTOR SEBI'S METHOD

T he Doctor achieved the cure of Herpes and HIV via detoxification and cleansing as his first method. He carefully detoxified the body at the intercellular and intracellular levels.

The detoxification and cleansing procedure involves the use of alkaline herbs that readily contain detoxifying and cleansing components. The detoxifying herbs help in detoxifying some organs in the body. He concluded that for the body to be clean of toxic substances, it must undergo detoxification. To eliminate any infection, disease, toxins, and excess acid from the body, it must initially undergo detoxification and cleansing. Therefore, Herpes and HIV are two viruses that attack the immune system. Hence, these viruses must be removed through intracellular and intercellular detoxification. Ultimately, Doctor Sebi generally detoxified the body off Herpes and HIV with the use of the same herbs and used other herbs for re-energizing the body to its normal state.

In other words, the treatment of both viruses involves:

Detoxification Process for HIV

Detoxification is very important in fighting against these viruses. The process involves engagement in fasting that might be very difficult for some individuals and very easy for others.

Doctor Sebi spoke about fasting for 70 days non-stop. Yes, it sounds scary, but it is possible for individuals who already enjoy fasting.

Fasting might be very difficult when you are engaging in it for the first time. However, you could get accustomed to it if you start gradually and adopt it with joy.

When you fast, the viruses attacking the immune system and CNS are stimulated and are removed via detoxification.

Your detoxification is perfectly completed with fasting within 14 days. Still, if you cannot fast, you can continue to take the herbs for a long period as the process of detoxification is reduced without fasting.

Therefore, the herbs required for proper detoxification are listed below:

- Burdock root

- Linden leaf

- Sea moss plant

- Elderberry

- Nettle root

The herbs used for detoxification help your body to perform the following functions:

- Removing toxic materials from the body.

- Multiplying cells in the body.

- Supplying the body with enough iron that is necessary for curing the herpes virus and HIV.

- Providing energy for the body.

- Re-energizing the body.

- Cleansing and promoting the blood and its vessels.

Caution

You can take some of the fruits listed in Doctor Sebi's recommended food list during your fast. Doctor Sebi took a lot of tamarind juice and water. Hence, you are required to drink about 4 liters of alkaline water daily and tamarind juice for proper detoxification.

You are likely going to get tired during this process. If you are tired or exhausted, take enough tamarind juice; it will increase your strength.

Do not miss dosages within the 14 days of detoxification as these viruses are capable of remaining dormant in the body. Still, if you continually take in the dosages and attack them accordingly, they will find their way out.

The above-listed herbs can make your poop beyond normal, so do not be afraid when you experience this. The poop is likely going to be watery, and you could visit the restroom about 4-6 times daily. When you discover that you visit the restroom too often above the specified times, take your bath and drink enough water.

Drinking enough water rehydrates you and helps ease these viruses and other toxic substances out of your body.

After the fasting is concluded, you are expected to start the next phase, regarded as the treatment phase. This involves the use of alkaline herbs to resuscitate the body and remove every leftover viral cell in the body.

Curing HIV: How Long Does It Take?

The weight and the health of an infected individual are the major factors to consider to know how long it requires for curing these viruses. This was declared by Doctor Sebi in one of his interviews.

Therefore, how long it takes to receive a cure for infected person A. might be different from infected person B. This is due to either the virus's stage, the weight of the sufferer, and the sufferer's health condition.

Additionally, the health state of the gut, liver, body fluids, and pancreas are some of the major factors that determine how long it takes a patient to achieve an absolute cure from this disease, he stated.

More so, he said, "Adopt fasting; plan and go for it. The more you fast, the quicker you receive your cure. You can consume dates if you are very weak in the process of fasting."

The Sebian Cure for HIV

There are different types of herbs that act as immunomodulators that help individuals suffering from HIV and AIDS. Examples of these herbs are:

- **Licorice:** The active ingredient in licorice is glycoside glycyrrhizin that acts as an immunomodulators and an antiviral agent, an ideal combination for addressing HIV infection. Intravenous glycyrrhizin has been employed for the treatment of individuals suffering from HIV infection in Japan since the 1980s. In early clinical trials, this therapy was very effective for suppressing HIV. Three long-term studies conducted in Japan have shown that oral administration of glycyrrhizin is also effective for maintaining immune function and suppressing HIV replication in an infected sufferer.

- **Dandelion:** it is reported that dandelion helps in preventing the replication and multiplication of the Human Immunodeficiency Virus (HIV) (Han et al. 2011). HIV replication is responsible for the advancement of Acquired Immunodeficiency Syndrome.

- **Echinacea (Coneflower):** This plant has been used at various times for the treatment of several health problems. It is a very common herb used by the Native Americans, and that are known to have immune-enhancing effects in humans. When white blood cells from individuals suffering from this infection are incubated with this plant, a definite stimulation of the white cells' activity is detected because the activity of the white cells is decreased in people infected with HIV. Therefore, this herb is an immune-enhancing herb that is extremely beneficial for individuals who have HIV and AIDS.

- **Reishi Mushroom:** this is one of the several fungal immunomodulators that have been used for thousands of years in Asia. Some data shows that the Reishi mushroom stimulates T-helper cells' activities taken from people who have HIV or AIDS. Several constituents have been identified in Reishi mushroom that are HIV protease inhibitors in vitro.

- Asian/American Ginseng

- Marshmallow

CHAPTER 14: DR. SEBI'S RECOMMENDED PRODUCTS THAT CAN HEAL THE HERPES SIMPLEX VIRUS

D r. Sebi recommended some effective natural herbal products that you can use to eradicate the herpes simplex virus from your body and become ultimately herpes free.

These natural herbal products include:

Pure Extract Giloy Tablet

Giloy tablets are obtained manually from high-quality giloy extracts. The giloy herb contains powerful antiviral properties that help to boost your immune system and fight viral infections such as the herpes simplex virus and sexually transmitted diseases.

Giloy contains powerful properties that can be useful to treat the herpes simplex virus and boost your health.

These properties are:

- Giloy extract is a potent antiviral agent.

- Giloy extract helps cold sores and blisters to heal faster.

- It helps to reduce inflammation.

- It helps to boost your immune system and help your body fight off infection.

AHP Zinc Powder

- AHP is also known as ayurvedic herbo purified. To get a high-quality AHP zinc powder, zinc is refined with natural purifying and detoxifying herbs such as Aloe Vera.

- AHP Zinc Powder is gotten from zinc that is created naturally, and this natural zinc is very easy for your body to absorb. Also, the naturally-occurring zinc is healthier than the usual off-counter zinc.

- AHP is very effective in treating the herpes virus, repairing damaged skin, and treating sores and blisters.

- The properties AHP Zinc Powder include:

- It helps to reduce and fight inflammation.

- It is instrumental in healing cold sores and wounds.

- It helps to heal skin infections.

- It promotes the healthy growth of your cells.

- it helps to boost your immune system and help your body to fight off diseases

- It contains powerful antiviral properties.

AHP Silver Powder

- Ayurvedically herbo purification is a process used to purify minerals in herbal mixtures to make them potent to heal infections and diseases.

- Ayurvedically herbo purification method ensures that the minerals are purified to improve the healing properties and absorb the healing properties of the herbal minerals used to purify it.

- AHP powder is very effective in treating disease conditions as the herpes virus, and Dr. Sebi administered this powder on many of his patients.

- AHP Silver Powder is very effective in treating the herpes simplex virus because it targets your nervous system, which is the hidden point of the infection in your body.

- The AHP Silver Powder performs the function of eradicating the herpes simplex virus from your body by sending silver nanoparticles into your nervous system to flush out the herpes virus.

- AHP Silver Powder contains potent and effective antiviral properties that enable it to treat cold sores, flu, and the herpes virus.

The properties of AHP Silver Powder include:

- It contains a potent antibacterial property that enables it to eradicate the herpes simplex virus from your body.

- It contains antibacterial properties.

- It helps to reduce inflammation that prevents the herpes simplex virus from healing.

- It quickens the healing of cold sores and blisters.

- It helps to eradicate skin infections.

Triphala

- Triphala is a powerful herb that contains three crucial herbal combinations. These herbal combinations are Behada, harda, and amla.

- Dr. Sebi recommended these three herbal combinations that make up the Triphala for the treatment of the herpes virus.

- Medical experts also acknowledged it because of its potency and efficacy.

- Dr. Sebi recommended this herbal combination for the eradication of the herpes virus from your body. These herbal combinations can also help purify and cleanse your body and remove toxins from your body and bloodstream.

The properties of the Triphala herb include:

- It helps to heal cold sores, blisters, and wounds.

- It is useful in reducing inflammation.

- It contains powerful antioxidants that quicken the healing of cold sores and blisters caused by the herpes virus.

- It contains powerful antiviral properties.

- It helps eradicate skin infections.

- It prevents bloating.

Purnarnavadi Mansoor

- Parnarnavadi Mandoor is a healthy and nutritious herbomineral that is prepared naturally from the combination of herbs, and not an ayurvedicallly herbo purified mineral.

- Purnarnavadi Mandoor is a combination of naturally occurring minerals such as iron, zinc, and calcium. It also contains powerful herbs like Alma, purnarnava, and shunti.

- The herbal combination contained in Purnarnavadi Mandoor is very effective in removing toxins from your body and cleansing your blood.

- Dr. Sebi recommends taking this herbal combination because he discovered that the liver function is disrupted during viral infection, thereby making healing impossible or slow. So the Purnarnavadi Mandoor helps to restore the liver to its normal function and quickens the healing process.

The properties of Purnarnavadi Mandoor include:

- It helps to reduce inflammation that blocks the healing process of the herpes simplex virus.

- It contains powerful antiviral properties that help to heal the herpes virus.

- It helps to heal blisters, cold sores, and wounds.

- It helps to eradicate skin infections and other infections in the body.

- It contains powerful antibacterial properties.

CHAPTER 15: OVERCOMING LUPUS WITH DR. SEBI

L upus is a horrible long-term autoimmune disease where your body's immune system gets hyperactive and begins to attack healthy, normal tissue. Some symptoms can include damage, swelling, and inflammation to your lungs, heart, blood, kidneys, skin, and joints.

Because of its complex nature, some people call lupus the "disease of 1,000 faces."

There are, on average, about 16,000 new cases of lupus every year in the United States. There are over one million people who are living with lupus. Lupus normally only affects women and happens between age 15 and 44.

In 2015, lupus gained attention when Selena Gomez announced she was diagnosed in her teen years and took treatments. Lupus isn't contagious, and it can't be transmitted in any way to another person. There have been extremely rare cases where a woman with lupus gave birth to a child who developed a lupus type. This is known as neonatal lupus.

Types of Lupus

There are several types of lupus. The main ones are neonatal, drug-induced, discoid, and systemic lupus erythematosus.

Neonatal

Most of the babies who are born to mothers who have systemic lupus erythematosus are usually healthy. About one percent of all the women who have autoantibodies related to lupus will give birth to a child with neonatal lupus.

The mother might have no symptoms of SLE. Sjogren's syndrome is another condition that can happen with lupus. Most of the symptoms include dry mouth and dry eyes.

If a baby is born with neonatal lupus, they might have low blood count, liver problems, or a skin rash. About ten percent have anemia. The rash will normally go away within a couple of weeks. Some infants will have a congenital heart block. This is when the heart can't regulate a rhythmic and normal pumping action. The baby might need to have a pacemaker. This could be a life-threatening condition.

If you have SLE and want to get pregnant, you need to talk with your doctor before and keep a close watch on yourself during your pregnancy.

Drug-Induced

About ten percent of all the people who have SLE will have symptoms that show up due to a reaction to specific drugs. There are about 80 drugs that can cause this condition.

These could include some drugs that are used to treat high blood pressure and seizures. They might include some oral contraceptives, antifungals, antibiotics, and thyroid medicines.

Some drugs that are associated with this type of lupus are:

- **Isoniazid:** this is an antibiotic that is used in the treatment for tuberculosis

- **Procainamide:** this is a medicine that is used to treat heart arrhythmias.

- **Hydralazine:** this is a medicine that is used to treat hypertension.

This type of lupus normally goes away once you stop taking the specific medication.

Discoid Lupus Erythematosus

With this type of lupus, the symptoms only affect the skin. Rashes will appear on the scalp, neck, and face. These areas might become scaly and thick, and scarring might happen. This rash could last from a couple of days to many years. If it does go away, it might come back.

DLE doesn't affect any internal organs, but about ten percent of all the people who have DLE will also develop SLE. It isn't clear if the people already had SLE, and it only showed up on the skin or if it progressed from DLE.

Systemic Lupus Erythematosus

This is a common type of lupus. This is a systemic condition, meaning that it can impact any part of the body. Symptoms could be anywhere from extremely mild to extremely severe.

This one is the most severe of all the types of lupus because it can affect any of the body's systems or organs. It could cause inflammation in the heart, blood, kidneys, lungs, joints, skin, or a combination of any of these.

This type of lupus normally goes through cycles. During remission times, the patient might not have any symptoms at all. When they have a flare-up, and the disease is very active, their symptoms will reappear.

Causes

We know that lupus is an autoimmune disease, but one exact cause hasn't been found.

Lupus happens when our immune systems attack healthy body tissues. It is more than likely that lupus is the result of a combination of your environment and genetics.

If a person has an inherited predisposition, they might develop lupus if they contact something in their environment that triggers lupus.

Our immune systems will protect our bodies and help to fight off antigens like germs, bacteria, and viruses. This happens because it produces proteins that are called antibodies. The B lymphocytes or white blood cells are what produce these antibodies.

If you have an autoimmune condition like lupus, your immune system can't tell the difference between healthy tissue, antigens, or unwanted substances. Because of this, our immune system will direct the antibodies to attack the antigens and healthy tissues. This can cause tissue damage, pain, and swelling.

An antinuclear antibody is the most common type of autoantibody that develops in people who have lupus. These ANA react with the cell's nucleus. All these autoantibodies are circulated throughout the blood, but some of the cells will have walls that are thin enough to allow some autoantibodies to move through them.

These autoantibodies could attack the body's DNA in the cells' nucleus. This is the reason why lupus will affect certain organs but not others.

Why Does the Immune System Go Wrong?

There are some genetic factors that play a role in the development of SLE. Some of the genes in the body can help the immune system to function properly. For people who have SLE, these changes could stop their immune system from working right.

One theory relates to the death of cells. This is a natural process that happens as the body renews cells. Some scientists think that because of some genetic factors, the body doesn't completely rid itself of all the dead cells. The cells that are dead and stay in the body might release substances that make the immune system malfunction.

Risk Factors

You might develop lupus due to many different factors. These could be environmental, genetic, hormonal, or any combination of these.

Environmental

Environmental agents like viruses or chemicals might contribute to causing lupus in certain people who might be genetically susceptible. Some possible environmental triggers could be:

- **Viral Infections:** These might trigger some symptoms in certain people who are susceptible to SLE.

- **Medications:** About ten percent of most cases of lupus could be related to a certain drug.

- **Sunlight:** Being exposed to sunlight can trigger lupus in some people.

- **Smoking:** The rise in more cases in the past several decades might be because of being exposed to tobacco.

Genetics

Scientists haven't proved that one certain genetic factor can cause lupus, even though it is a lot more common in some families.

Genetics might be the cause of the following risk factors:

Family History. Anyone who has a first or second-degree relative who has lupus will have a higher risk of getting lupus. Scientists have found specific genes that might contribute to getting lupus. There just hasn't been enough evidence to prove that they actually cause the disease.

In some studies done with identical twins, one twin might get lupus while the other doesn't, even if they did grow up together and have been exposed to the same environmental factors. If one twin has lupus, the other one will have about a 25 percent chance of getting this disease, too. Identical twins are more genetically imposed to have this condition.

Lupus could happen to people who don't have any family history of this disease, but there might be other autoimmune diseases within the family. Some examples include idiopathic thrombocytopenic purpura, hemolytic anemia, and thyroiditis.

Some researchers think that changes to the X-chromosomes might increase the risk.

Race. People of a certain background can develop lupus, but it is about three times more common in people who have an African background as compared to Caucasians. It is also more prevalent in Native American, Asian, and Hispanic women.

Hormones

These are chemicals that get produced by the body. They help to regulate and control activities of certain organs or cells.

This hormonal activity might explain these risk factors:

Age. The diagnosis and symptoms usually happen between the ages of 15 and 45, basically, during a woman's childbearing years. But about 20 percent of all cases happen after a woman turns 50.

Since nine out of ten lupus diagnoses are female, scientists have looked at a link between lupus and estrogen. Women and men produce estrogen, but women do produce more.

In one study done in 2016, some scientists found that estrogen could affect the immune activity and cause lupus antibodies to develop in women who are more susceptible to lupus.

This could explain who autoimmune disease will affect more women than men. In 2010, scientists published a study that reported women who had been diagnosed with lupus reported more fatigue and pain when menstruating. This might suggest that symptoms might flare more during this time.

There just isn't enough evidence that will confirm that estrogen actually causes lupus. If there is an actual link, an estrogen-based treatment could regulate how severe lupus gets. A lot more research is needed before doctors offer it as an actual treatment.

Gut Microbiota. Researchers have recently been looking at gut microbiota as one factor in developing lupus. Scientists say specific changes to gut microbiota happened in both mice and people who have lupus. They need more research in this area.

Can Children Be At Risk?

Lupus is very rare in children who are under 15 years of age if their birth mother didn't have it. If their birth mother had it, they might have lupus-related skin, liver, or heart problems.

Infants who have neonatal lupus might have higher chances of getting a different autoimmune disease later in their life.

Symptoms

During flare-ups is when people who have lupus will feel the symptoms. People with lupus will not have any or will only have a few symptoms in between flare-ups.

Lupus has many symptoms, and these include:

- Arthritis

- Purple or pale toes or finger from stress or cold

- Unusual hair loss

- Chest pain when taking deep breaths

- Headaches

- Fever

- Sensitive to sun

- Mouth ulcers

- Skin rashes caused by bleeding under the skin

- Swollen lymph nodes or glands

- Swelling around the eyes or in the legs

- Swelling or pain in the muscles or joints

- Weight loss and a loss of appetite

- Fatigue

CHAPTER 16: DR. SEBI'S HERBS FOR HAIR GROWTH AND HAIR PROBLEMS

Hair loss is a problem that affects both men and women frequently, and it is accumulating over the years. Hair loss is most common in men as they experience complete baldness. However, women also experience hair loss through hair thinning, weakness, breakage, and falling off.

Hair loss could be corrected through the employment of Dr. Sebi's alkaline herbs and diets. Therefore, the herbs that are effective for hair growth and are capable of fighting hair loss will be discussed in this chapter.

The following are Dr. Sebi's recommended herbs for hair growth and hair abnormalities treatment:

- **Marshmallow root:** It is rich in proteins and vitamins. It helps in the treatment of hair problems such as eczema, psoriasis, and dry scalp. It helps with the mucilage, which is a gel-like substance that becomes slippery when wet. It also helps in softening hair and helps in improving healthy hair growth.

- **Nettle:** It helps in alleviating hair loss through the stimulation of the scalp, improves blood circulation, and protects against further damage and breakage of the hair.

- **Licorice:** It helps in moisturizing the scalp and hydrating the hair. This herb also prevents and fights many common hair problems such as dandruff, scabs, and itching. This herb can also be helpful in fighting baldness and improve hair growth.

- **Dandelion:** This herb is rich in vitamin A, magnesium, iron, potassium, phosphorus, calcium, choline, and more. These nutrients are effective in improving hair growth through the treatment of the scalp and follicles.

- **Saw palmetto:** This herb is used for the treatment of hair loss.

- **Watercress:** It is rich in Vitamin A, biotin, and potassium. This makes it an excellent herb for hair loss, it helps active hair growth, nourishes the hair shaft, and supports the growth of fresh hair.

- **Flaxseed:** It is rich in fatty acids that are essential for your hair and antioxidants that remove free radicals. It nourishes the hair, strengthens the hair, prevents hair loss, and soothes the hair.

- **Coconut oil:** It helps in facilitating hair growth. Coconut oil is important in protecting the hair scalp and gives you smooth, shiny, and soft hair. This oil is also essential in preventing and fighting splitting and broken hair through strengthening the hair.

- **Sage:** It contains antiseptic and astringent components that help in promoting longer, fuller, thicker, and shiny hair.

- Olive oil

- Thyme

Preparation of the Herbs

1. Rinse, dry, and grind the following herbs together dandelion, saw palmetto, sage, nettle, marshmallow, licorice, watercress, and flaxseed.

2. Collect half tsp. of each herb and add into two cups of water.

3. Boil for about five minutes.

4. Drain and drink two times daily.

5. You can collect half tsp. of each herb and boil with three cups of water.

Use this to wash your hair once a day.

1. Collect two tbsp. of undiluted coconut oil and two tbs. of olive oil.

2. Add two tbsp. of powdered thyme and curry herbs.

3. Mix thoroughly and apply to your hair.

4. You can add the mixture to your hair cream and apply it thoroughly.

Non-Dr. Sebi's Herbs For Hair Growth And Hair Problems

Some other herbs are effective for improving hair growth and fighting hair abnormalities. These herbs are regarded as non-Dr. Sebi's herbs.

These non-Dr. Sebi's herbs are:

- **Aloe Vera:** The constant usage of this plant's gel on hair helps in sustaining the pH of the hair. It helps in making the scalp conditioned and also improves hair health. It facilitates opening up the obstructed pores in the scalp and increases hair follicles' growth, thereby improving hair growth.

- **Sesame:** Sesame oil is rich in vitamins, omega fatty acids, and all nutrients necessary for hair growth and hair abnormalities. This oil is important for improving hair health through fighting hair problems such as ringworm, dandruff, head lice, dryness, psoriasis, and more. Sesame oil prevents hair and scalp exposure from U.V light. Constant use of sesame oil may cause your hair to become dark; hence, this oil is beneficial for individuals growing gray hair.

- **Almond oil:** This oil is loaded with Vitamin A and E. Almond oil is very effective in fighting scalp infections and inflammation, and many other hair problems.

- **Ginseng:** This is another natural herb that helps in preventing and fighting hair loss. It increases the transfer of blood from the bloodstream to the scalp, thereby ensuring the hair follicles receive enough blood and nutrition, giving way for healthy and strong hair. It is very effective in combating baldness and helps hair growth.

- **Neem:** Neem leave is very effective for improving hair and scalp health. This plant helps in increasing the easy supply of blood through the blood vessel to the scalp. When this happens, hair is expected to grow quickly, thus, preventing hair loss and untimely hair gray.

- **Rosemary:** Have you heard about any herb that is capable of detoxifying the hair scalp? Rosemary is a special herb that can help you do that. Because when you detoxify your scalp, it helps you prevent hair loss and hair abnormalities. Rosemary helps in making your hair stronger, especially your hair root.

- **Amla (Indian Gooseberry):** This herb is rich in vitamins C, B complex, iron, calcium, and more. It is used very widely for treating hair loss in India. Amla does many functions for your hair when used regularly: it conditions and strengthens the hair and also promotes hair growth.

- **Chinese Hibiscus:** This is a powerful herb that helps in preventing premature greying of the hair, and it also promotes hair growth. Many hair problems are managed with the use of this herb.

- **Moringa:** This plant is very effective in providing strength for the hair follicles and helps in preventing hair from falling out. Moringa is also used as a natural conditioner and facilitates hair growth.

- **Lavender:** Lavender oil contains antibacterial, antimicrobial, antiseptic, and anti-inflammatory components. It is essential in fighting baldness, increasing hair growth, and improves hair health. His oil helps in fighting hair and scalp problems such as head lice, dandruff, dry scalp, and many other scalp infections. The constant use of this oil assists in preventing hair from falling off and facilitates rapid hair growth. You can use this oil by applying it on your scalp and hair and massage very well to ensure penetration of the oil on the hair.

How To Use Sesame Oil, Almond Oil, And Aloe Vera Gel

This mixture is very effective for fighting the above-mentioned hair problems as well as improving hair growth.

1. Collect about one tbsp. of sesame oil, almond oil, and add the same proportion of Aloe Vera gel.

2. Place on a pan that is capable of heating the mixture.

3. Allow the mixture to heat properly for about 2 minutes.

4. Allow it to get cool slightly and apply on your scalp massaging thoroughly.

5. Allow it to stay on your hair for about 40 minutes.

6. Rinse with shampoo.

Now, here is another treatment you can use with the remaining herbs:

Preparation

- Rinse, dry, and grind the following herbs Ginseng, Neem, Rosemary, Amla (Indian Gooseberry), Chinese Hibiscus, and Moringa separately.

- Collect a half tsp. of each herb and add into two cups of water.

- Boil for about five minutes.

- Drain and drink two times daily.

- On the other hand, you can collect half tsp. of each herb and boil with three cups of water.

Use this to wash your hair once a day.

CHAPTER 17: HAIR LOSS DOESN'T HAVE TO BE PERMANENT

Alopecia or hair loss is a problem for children, women, and men. Treatments include hair restoration techniques, hair replacements, or medicines like Rogaine and Propecia.

Hair is made from a protein known as keratin. This is made in the hair follicles on the outer layer of our skin. When the follicles make new hair, the old gets pushed out of the skin's surface at a rate of six inches each year. Most of the time, around 90 percent of the hair on your head will be growing. Every follicle has its own individual life cycle that gets influenced by disease, age, and other factors. This cycle can be divided into three phases:

- **Anagen:** This phase will last about two to six years. This is when the hair is actively growing.

- **Catagen:** This phase will only last about two or three weeks. This is a period of transitional hair growth.

- **Telogen:** This phase will last around two or three months. This is a time of rest. When this phase is over, the old hair is shed, and new hair will replace it. The cycle begins all over again.

When people begin aging, their hair growth rate will slow down. There are several types of hair loss:

- **Scarring Alopecias:** This can result in permanent hair loss. Acne, folliculitis, and cellulitis, which are all inflammatory skin conditions among other disorders like lichen planus and lupus, can cause scars that will get rid of the hair's ability to regenerate. Hair that is woven too tightly and using hot instruments that pull on the hair can cause permanent hair loss.

- **Telogen Effluvium:** Many hairs go into a resting phase at one time, this causes the hair to shed and then thin.

- **Trichotillomania:** This is mostly seen in small children. It is a psychological disorder where they pull out their own hair.

- **Alopecia Universalis:** This can cause all the hair on the body to fall out, including pubic hair, eyelashes, and eyebrows.

- **Alopecia Areata:** It usually begins all of a sudden and can cause some patchy hair loss in young adults and children. This could cause total baldness or alopecia totalis. Around 90 percent of everyone who has this condition has their hair come back in a couple of years.

- **Androgenic Alopecia:** This is a condition that is genetic and can affect women and men. Men who have this condition that we call male pattern baldness could begin losing their hair in their teens or early 20s. It can be seen by a receding hairline with a gradual disappearance of hair from the front of the scalp and the crown. Women who have this problem that we call female pattern baldness won't notice this thinning until they reach their 40s or even later in life.

- **Involutional Alopecia:** This is a condition that is natural where the hair gradually gets thinner with age. More of the hair follicles will enter into the resting stage. This makes the rest of the hairs get fewer in number and shorter.

Causes of Hair Loss

No one actually knows why some hair follicles have been programmed to have shorter growth cycles than others. There are several factors that can influence hair loss:

- **Diet:** A diet that severely restricts calories or protein could cause hair loss. If you aren't getting enough protein, your body might ration out the protein in your body by shutting down your hair growth.

- **Medical conditions:** Anemia, eating disorders, iron deficiency anemia, diabetes, lupus, and thyroid disease could all cause hair loss. Most of the time, once the condition gets treated, the hair will return as long as there wasn't any scarring from follicular disorders, lichen planus, or lupus. Anemia happens because of an iron deficiency and can cause hair loss. Your doctor can do a blood test to make sure you have anemia. Taking an iron supplement could fix this problem. Hypothyroidism is basically an underactive thyroid. This small gland that is located in your neck makes hormones that are needed for your metabolism along with your development and growth. If it isn't pumping enough hormones into your body, it can cause hair loss.

- **Cosmetic procedures:** Dyeing your hair, bleaching, perms, and shampooing excessively can cause your hair to thin because it makes the hair brittle and weak. Using hot curlers or rollers, braiding your hair too tight, and running a pick through very tight curls could break and damage hair

- **Autoimmune disease:** Most autoimmune diseases could cause alopecia areata. This type of baldness causes the immune system to crank up for reasons unknown and can affect the hair follicles. In some of the people who have alopecia areata, their hair will grow back, even though it might be very fine and a lighter color than before. The normal thickness and color will eventually return.

- **Age:** It isn't uncommon to notice that your hair is thinning once you reach 50 years of age. This type of hair loss can't be treated unless you want to undergo hair transplants. Using scarves and wigs is one way to go.

- **X-rays, injuries, and burns:** Any of these could cause a temporary hair loss. In these cases, your normal hair will return when the injury has healed unless it produces a scar. If this happens, the hair won't ever return.

- **Pulling your hair:** One impulse control disorder called trichotillomania can cause you to pull out your hair. You don't have any control over it, you just constantly pull and play with your hair. This can cause big chunks of your hair to fall out.

- **Drugs:** There are specific classes of drugs that can cause hair loss. The most common are beta-blockers that are used to treat blood pressure and some blood thinners. Other drugs that could cause hair loss are antidepressants, ibuprofen, and other NSAIDs, lithium, and methotrexate.

- **Childbirth:** It is a good example of physical stress that can cause you to lose your hair. This is more common after you have given birth because having a baby is traumatic. If you do lose your hair after you give birth, don't worry because your hair will come back in a few months.

- **Stress and illness:** Any type of trauma, like an illness, car accident, or surgery, could cause hair loss. This hair loss happens when stress causes the hair roots to be pushed into the resting or shedding stages. This is just temporary, and your hair will begin to grow back once your body recovers.

- **Vitamin A:** Taking too much vitamin A could trigger your hair loss. The normal daily value for Vitamin A is about 5,000 IU each day. Taking more than 10,000 IU daily could cause you to lose your hair. This is completely reversible. Just stop taking vitamin A.

- **Deficient in Vitamin B:** This isn't common in the United States; having a deficiency of vitamin B can cause hair loss. You can also change up your diet. Vitamin B can be found in fruits other than citrus, starchy vegetables, meat, and fish. Eating a balance of vegetables and fruits along with "good fats" like nuts and avocado are good for your health and hair.

- **Quick weight loss:** Suddenly losing weight is a type of trauma that could cause you to lose your hair. The weight loss can put some unnecessary stress on your body. Since you haven't been eating right, it could have resulted in mineral or vitamin deficiencies. Losing your hair and weight might be a sign of eating disorders like bulimia or anorexia. This, too, will fix itself with some time. You will have about six months of hair loss, and then it will come back.

- **Genes:** If you come from a long line of hair loss, you are going to have it, too. Inheriting genes from both the female and male parent could influence a predisposition to getting female or male pattern baldness.

- **Anabolic Steroids:** If you are taking steroids to bulk up, you might find that your hair begins to fall out. These have the same impact on your body the PCOS does. Your hair should return once you stop taking the steroids.

- **Hormones:** Just like the pregnancy hormone can cause hair loss, if you stop taking your birth control pill, this can cause it, too. The change of hormone that happens during menopause could cause the same thing. An abnormal level of androgens, which are male hormones that are produced by both women and men, can cause hair loss.

Signs of Hair Loss

These signs will vary between children, women, and men. But people of any sex or age might notice some more hair being collected in your shower drain or hairbrush.

Some signs of hair loss in men might include:

- A semi-circle shaped pattern that exposes the crown

- Receding hairline

- Thinner hair

Signs of hair loss in women:

- Thinning of the hair, especially at the crown

Signs of hair loss in young adults and children:

- Excessive shedding of hair after stress, anemia, rapid weight loss, drug treatments, and illnesses

- Incomplete hair loss or patches of broken hairs on the eyebrows or scalp

- Total loss of hair over all the body

- Sudden loss of hair in patches

- When to call your doctor:

- Your child or yourself have suffered an unexplained hair loss on any body part

- Your child is pulling or rubbing out their hair

- Your child has incomplete hair loss or broken hairs on their eyebrows or scalp

- Your child or yourself has a sudden loss of hair in patches

Treatments

There are some remedies that promise to restore hair to a balding head, and some of these have been used since ancient times. Most women and men who have thinning hair can't do much to reverse this process. Most people will turn to weaving, hairpieces, and wigs after they lost their hair from drug treatments or surgery. Some people could benefit from these treatments:

- Janus Kinase Inhibitors: This is a class of immunomodulators and its results in clinical studies that treat alopecia areata are promising.

- Lasers: Home-based and office laser devices have been successful in stimulating hair growth.

- Diphencyprone: This is a sensitizing agent that is used topically and only occasionally to stimulate the hair growth for people who have alopecia areata.

- Anthralin or Drithocreme: This is a medication that is used topically to control the inflammation around the base of the hair follicles. It has been used to treat conditions like alopecia areata.

Prevention

Even though there isn't a total cure for balding, you could protect your hair from being damaged and leading to the thinning of the hair.

In order to prevent damage to your hair, do the following:

- **Brush right:** Not brushing your hair properly could do the same damage to your hair as any other product. Using the right brush, apply gentle pressure to the scalp and bring the brush down to the tips of the hair to distribute the natural oils into the hair. You have to work gently and don't brush your hair when it is wet. This is the time when your hair is most fragile. When your hair is wet, you need to use a wide-tooth comb.

- **Pick the right products:** Use a shampoo that is right for your type of hair. If you like curling your hair, pick sponge rollers as they won't damage your hair. Use a natural-bristle brush that is slightly stiff. It won't break or tear the hair.

- **Be natural:** Try to leave your hair its natural texture and color. If this isn't an option, give your hair time to recover between chemical treatments or blowouts. Don't tightly braid your hair.

CHAPTER 18: PRECAUTIONS REGARDING PH BALANCE & THE ALKALINE DIET

When beginning any diet or new eating habits, some important factors consider when choosing the alkaline diet. First, determine if you have any health conditions that could be impacted by a change in your pH levels. For most, if not all, health conditions, an alkaline diet is one of the best plans to follow, though it's always a good idea to clear any potential medical professional issues. If you have allergies or food sensitivities, this could be caused by a temporary sensitivity or effect of a condition that may be resolved through a change in diet. If the food(s) you have an allergic reaction to happen to be acidic, then the solution is as simple as eliminating them from your diet. If the food item is more alkaline, it can be substituted for an alternative until the sensitivity disappears or changes altogether.

When adapting to an alkaline-based meal plan, always note your body's reaction to certain foods and combinations of foods. Even when you reduce the acidity level in your diet, avoid adding too much sugar or salt to your foods. Fruits have their natural sugar, fructose, which is easily digested and used by the body, unlike processed or artificial sweeteners. Salt is good as long as we get the required amount through our diet, though adding too much can elevate blood pressure and contribute to hypertension.

Unless you have severe allergies or must avoid certain foods due to conflicts with medication or other medical conditions, the alkaline diet is a very nutritious way to eat. By planning your meals carefully, you can ensure that all nutrient requirements are met and avoid deficiencies. General guidelines to take into consideration when beginning the alkaline diet are fairly easy to follow:

- Drink plenty of water. If eight glasses a day is too much to strive for, then drink natural teas and sparkling water.

- Keep track of any adverse reactions during your diet. If your body reacts in a negative way, such as indigestion or high blood pressure, it could be that some of the foods you are selecting may not be as alkaline as perceived.

- Stay active. This is a good idea regardless of the diet you follow, as exercise prevents many conditions, improves cardiovascular function, heart health, and increases oxygen levels in your body.

- Make small changes at first to incorporate alkaline foods into your diet without making a drastic overhaul of your diet. This will allow your body to become adjusted to the new types of foods you'll be getting used to over some time.

How to Achieve Permanent Results?

The alkaline diet can produce very positive results on your health and well-being. If you suffer from chronic pain and conditions associated with a highly acidic environment, this way of eating will provide substantial relief. The success of your diet determines how well and consistent it is followed and incorporated into your lifestyle. Some people consider dieting as a temporary, and once you achieve a specific goal or level of weight loss or a similar result, they switch back to their previous food choices. To achieve permanent results, consistency in the way you eat, exercise, and live is essential in maintaining good health. Incorporating alkaline foods into your everyday meals and food options is the best way to meet your goals and maintain the benefit of a healthy lifestyle indefinitely.

Keeping a consistently healthy and budget-friendly shopping list that includes a roster of your favorite alkaline foods is a good way to stay on track. If you find yourself leaning towards more acidic food options, weigh the benefits of incorporating the food items into your current diet, or find a suitable substitute, if possible. Once your body grows accustomed to alkaline foods, you'll notice a shift in your cravings and what you enjoy. This is a positive change that indicates your body is adjusting to a new set of "rules" for eating, and over time, this will become routine and easy.

CHAPTER 19: SUPPLEMENTS TO TAKE DAILY

The very best approach to acquire the critical substances you desire (minerals, vitamins, essential fatty acids, fats -- the list continues on and on) is via a balanced, healthful, nutritional supplement (one which is 100 percent natural if possible). However, the truth is that a number of individuals have quite a difficult time eating enough of the ideal sorts of foods to acquire the materials they require in the right amounts. That is why it is highly suggested that you carefully think about using nutritional supplements to improve the quantities of crucial stuff your body needs to have to work at its best.

It might appear overwhelming to consider carrying ten (or more) distinct supplements daily but remember that doing this could be a true advantage to your body and head. Additionally, it might allow you to stay longer and much healthier. Nevertheless, if you are aware that you are getting a fantastic amount of a few of these chemicals in your diet plan and you are interested in maintaining the number of supplements you are taking comparatively low, you can correct your nutritional regimen so. For example, if you consume lots of fatty, cold-water fish, then you might not have to supplement using omega-3 fatty acids. Consider your daily diet and nutritional supplement in a proper method to ensure you're giving your body exactly what it requires.

Here is one important note to remember while you're considering nutritional supplements: Your daily recommended allowances for vitamins, minerals, nutritional supplements, and other chemicals that you see on food labels do not indicate a great deal. These tips show you the minimum quantities necessary for the body to keep working properly. However, they do not let you know exactly what amounts you will need for the body to really go beyond and above that foundation level.

Multivitamin

Some people today choose a once-a-day multivitamin. While that is definitely better than simply taking nothing in any way, the tablet likely does not include things large enough dosages of all the vitamins that you want. How can I know? If a once-a-day vitamin comprised adequately substantial doses of 14 essential vitamins, then it might need to be as large as a golf club. The majority of the multivitamins offering comprehensive vitamin policy ask that you take a few pills every day. Four capsules or tablets per day is a fairly typical number.

A variety of great brands and moderately priced options can be found. You would like to locate an organization that does third party analysis. Most of their better products aren't offered across the counter and have to be bought via an undercover doctor or a drugstore involved in natural well-being. Guarantee that the multivitamin you select includes a great calcium source, and be certain it functions as calcium hydroxylapatite rather than calcium carbonate. You do not automatically have to realize the differences between both; simply ensure your multivitamin involves the former rather than the latter.

Multimineral

In general, you will need to provide your system using 16 distinct nutritional supplements if you would like it to perform in an optimum level.

Multi-mineral nutritional supplements are simple to discover, and in several instances, you are able to discover multivitamin/multi-mineral combination nutritional supplements. These options can be challenging, and you have to be certain if you decide to go that path, you purchase an option that comprises all 14 vitamins along with all of 16 nutritional supplements. (That is rather a good deal!)

If you are picking a multi-mineral supplement, then go with one which features chelated minerals. I will spare you all of the dull details of this procedure, which produces chelated minerals. But remember that unless you are getting chelated minerals, then you are likely paying for nutritional supplements that wind up on your bathroom rather than on your own body's major systems.

Do not choose a multi-mineral supplement that arrives out of a clay resource. These goods aren't chelated, plus they feature tin, silver, and nickel. Sometimes they even record lead as a component!

Omega-3 Fatty Acids

You have probably read or heard regarding omega-3 fatty acids in the news lately. The significance of this essential fatty acid was getting a great deal of press, also for great reason. It is one of these substances your body needs to endure and flourish. Despite all of the wonderfully intricate chemical processes that your own body can perform, it cannot fabricate omega-3 fatty acids.

The best dietary source of omega-3s is beef. Fish is another great resource. You ought to consume fish as part of a proper diet; however, unless you are eating wild Alaskan salmon, or even among those other few kinds of fish which do not commonly contain elevated levels of mercury, it is likely that you're becoming an extremely salty dose of toxins with your own omega-3 fatty acids.

To stay clear of germs but nevertheless get your omega-3 supplement, use liquid fish oil or even some capsule or soft gel. Take 1 g twice per day to get exactly what you want.

Resveratrol

Resveratrol is a highly effective antioxidant, and I recommend that everybody get a dose of this every day. Resveratrol has generated a higher profile as a Harvard Medical School case study. A couple of years back it was revealed that a fairly dramatic gain in mice's health and lifespan after they have been given resveratrol. Should you read up about this particular antioxidant, you're likely going to see it is in red wine, which is the reality. However, if you wished to receive an important dose of resveratrol from red wine, you'd need to glug a couple of hundred bottles of the material daily, which will kill you before you have to enjoy the advantages of resveratrol.

The fantastic thing is you can purchase resveratrol supplements in many health food shops and in any vitamin store, either in person or on the internet. You will find it labeled either as resveratrol or red wine extract. I suggest getting 30 mg every day that ought to be somewhat simple, given the width of nutritional supplements options available on the industry.

Vitamin C

If you choose a fantastic multivitamin, then you are likely to get a fantastic amount of vitamin C every day. But do not believe for a moment you are getting all your body should truly have the ability to work on a top degree.

I suggest carrying a 1,000-milligram vitamin C supplement two times every day. I know that seems like a great deal, but if you've read about it, you understand why I believe very strongly that vitamin C is a massive blessing for your great health. Though it's within plenty of vegetables and fruits, it may continue to be hard to get enough of the things on your diet plan. Hundreds (maybe thousands) of vitamin C supplement options are available, so do some research and speak with your naturopathic physician to discover which ones are ideal for you.

If you are fighting a disease, take 8,000 mg of vitamin C daily rather than the normal 2,000 mg.

Vitamin B Complex

The term vitamin B complex describes all of the B vitamins: B1, B2, B3, B5, B6, B7, B9, and B12. A number of the B vitamins also have several other widely used titles – riboflavin and niacin are just two great examples.

The assortment of important features the vitamin B complex performs on the human body is shocking, and I would not even try to cover all of the details. Just know that in the event you would like to be healthy and live a long, comfy lifestyle, you had better concentrate on getting lots of B vitamins.

It's a fantastic idea to have a vitamin B complex supplement as well as a multivitamin daily. You'll be able to discover such a supplement that can provide you exactly what you need in just one dose every day.

Magnesium

Several strong studies performed over the past couple of years have demonstrated very powerful connections between elevated levels of magnesium intake and the avoidance of cardiovascular disease. Individuals who get lots of calcium – within their diets and during supplementing – normally possess a reduced heart disease risk. Additionally, magnesium is also involved in approximately 300 different biochemical reactions that happen within your own body, which means that you may see why it is a fantastic idea to be certain that you're getting enough. To be sure, have a supplement which provides you 600 mg each day.

Sulforaphane

Not everybody has heard of sulforaphane, and that is too bad. It has been making headlines on a fairly regular basis recently, and everybody ought to be carrying it as a nutritional supplement regularly.

Recent studies have suggested that sulforaphane will help thwart some sorts of cancer and may slow tumor growth. Additional studies reveal that sulforaphane lessens the quantity of H. pylori bacteria from the gut, which is what triggers stomach lining inflammation and nausea. If those are not good reasons to choose sulforaphane every day, I do not understand what exactly they are.

You're able to get sulforaphane in supplement form in 2 manners: carrot seed infusion or plain sulforaphane. If you go for the latter, then take for 500 mg daily. In case the prior is the favorite sulforaphane nutritional supplement, attempt to receive 30 mg daily.

Vitamin E

Along with vitamin C and vitamin B complex, vitamin E is something which will almost surely be included on your multivitamin routine but likely not in large enough quantities. You'll be able to see continuing health benefits of supplementing with vitamin E around 800 mg every day, and therefore don't be reluctant to take that much.

What are a few of the health advantages of taking extra vitamin E? To begin with, vitamin E has strong antioxidant effects. But vitamin E does a number of other fantastic things for the body too, from boosting your immune system to maintaining blood vessels at tiptop form.

Do yourself massive favor, and do not scrimp on the vitamin E.

Alpha-Lipoic Acid (ALA)

You will frequently see the lipoic acid known as ALA. It is a top-notch antioxidant that helps your body fight infection and retains your cells working at a higher level.

Choose an ALA nutritional supplement and locate a capsule type that produces about 800 mg every day. That amount was demonstrated to provide many health benefits with no overpowering or side-effects within the human body. It's possible to locate ALA supplements in any fantastic health food shop and in the regional vitamin retailer.

CHAPTER 20: CLASSIFICATION OF FOODS

Foods are classified into different forms, depending on whether they contain acids and alkaline. Examples of foods are hybridized food, raw foods, live food, Genetically Modified Foods (GMO), drugs, and dead foods.

Hybridized Foods

They are foods that are not natural. They are created and formed by cross-pollination. The vitamins and mineral levels cannot be quantified, and they cannot be grown naturally.

Foods that are cross-pollinated (hybridized) lack the proper mineral balance that is present in wild foods. Consumption of hybridized foods results in a lack (deficiency) of minerals in the body.

Fruits and vegetables that are hybridized result in excessive stimulation of the body, which subsequently results in loss of minerals in the body.

It is reported that hybridized foods lack electrically charged components. This is because most soils in the world, especially the United States, lack minerals, thereby affecting the foods that are planted on them as long as the soil lack minerals, the crops planted on them will automatically lack minerals.

This implies that most foods we eat daily are junk. Junks foods are reported to be void of nutrition, and this results in several health problems.

Hybrid foods are mostly sugars that cannot be identified by the body's digestive system. Examples are cows, pigs, watermelon, chicken, sausage roll, and many others.

The engineers that are involved in producing hybridized foods always conclude that they are doing it for individual to get enough food for consumption but unknowingly, they are causing us more harm than good.

Raw Foods

Raw foods are living foods that have not undergone processing, and they are uncooked. They are foods that are dried with the use of direct sunlight and are majorly organic foods.

When raw foods are eaten, there is a high tendency that the individual loses weight because it helps the digestive system to quickly digest the foods. This implies that raw foods are beneficial for those who have the intention of losing weight and are ready to keep lean and clean.

These foods also contain many components needed for the digestion process and are destroyed within a short time if not properly dried.

Raw foods help in the improvement of overall health and can help in fighting against disease-causing organisms. Many individuals that inculcate the habit of eating raw food spend little or no money in the hospital because their immune system is competent.

However, other dieters believe that raw foods could contain poison that might cause harm to the body. They, therefore, advise that raw foods should be cooked to remove some toxic substances in it. Such foods include undercooked meat, chicken, fish and more. They concluded that cooking food helps in killing every viable bacterial and other disease-causing organisms that may be present in them.

Live Foods

Live foods are foods that are not dead without consuming them. All live foods do not contain toxic components when they are left to undergo fermentation.

They are foods that are not processed, cooked, microwaved, irradiated, genetically modified, drenched with chemicals (pesticides, insecticides, and preservatives).

Moreso, living foods do not undergo destruction when they are not in their environment. The materials required for the process of digestion are embedded in living food, which contains almost the same pH with water.

Live foods are foods that can restore the micro-electrical potential of the cells in the body.

Therefore, live foods help the body to become re-energized and cause it to be in the state that is fit to fight any disease. It is also important in detoxifying the body in the intercellular and intracellular level.

Genetically Modified Foods (GMO)

These are food improved by the man with the use of genetics. They mostly damage the immunity in the body. These foods form an abnormal approach in humans and also cause genetic consequence in the body.

Genetically modified foods contain genes of allergen, which facilitates allergic reactions in the body. Excess consumption of Genetically Modified Foods is reported to be associated with the inability to resist bacteria in the body.

Examples are foods that are grown hastily, weather-resistant foods such as corn, yeast, brown rice, and many others.

Drugs

Many drugs are dangerous and harmful to the body. They are extremely toxic and acidic. Most of them are extracted and are synthetic.

Drugs can influence and affect several body organs, thereby reducing the immune system, increasing the susceptibility of infections and diseases, as well as causing cardiovascular problems.

Examples are cocaine, sugar, all prescription drugs, heroin, and many others.

Dead Foods

These are foods that, when fermented, become toxic, and they have a prolonged life span. They are overdone and over-processed foods.

Dead foods are associated with the risk of having depression, cancer, untimely death, cardiovascular diseases and problems, poor digestion, and diabetes. Dead foods facilitate the accumulation of fatty tissues in the body, which could result in the aforementioned health problems. Dead food is void of nutrients because the refining process has taken almost all the nutrients (fibers, vitamins, minerals) available in it.

Most of the dead foods are so tasty and inviting that you continue eating them without stopping. As a result, you become fat and feel sick.

Examples are deep-fried foods, synthetic foods, white rice, sugar, soft drinks, snacks, desserts, alcohols, sugars, and many more.

CHAPTER 21: 8 ALKALINE FOODS YOU SHOULD INCLUDE IN YOUR DAILY DIET

Alkaline foods assist in countering the potential risks of acidity and acidity refluxes, bringing some kind of relief. The majority of traditional Indian foods contain alkaline foods to make a balanced diet.

If you focused on your chemistry lessons at school, you'll be acquainted with the idea of acidity and alkali. If not really, then here is a quick review: Acids are essentially aqueous solutions that have a pH degree of significantly less than 7.0, whereas alkalis possess a pH degree of a lot more than 7.0, drinking water being the natural component having a pH of 7.0. In simpler conditions, acids are sour in flavor and corrosive in character, whereas alkalis are components that neutralize acids.

During digestion, our stomach secretes gastric acids that assist in wearing down food. The stomach includes its own pH, which varies from 2.0 to 3.5, which is highly acidic but essential for the procedure of digestion. Nevertheless, sometimes, because of an unhealthy way of life and food practices, the stomach's acidic level goes haywire, resulting in acidity, acidity refluxes, and additional gastric ailments. Things that are acidic in character when digested by your body are meat, milk products, eggs, certain whole grains, processed sugars, and processed foods. It's important to note an ingredient's acidity or alkaline-developing tendency in the stomach has nothing in connection with the real pH of the meals itself.

Citric fruits are acidic in character, but citric acidity actually comes with an alkalizing impact inside our body.

Alkaline foods are essential in order to bring in stability. Like all specialists and doctors have already been saying for a long time, we should possess a well-balanced meal with an excellent mixture of everything, instead of restraining ourselves from possessing only a particular category of foods. Alkaline foods consequently assist in countering the potential risks of acidity and acidity refluxes, bringing some kind of relief. Many traditional Indian foods contain alkaline foods to make a well-balanced diet. If you've ever tried an average Assamese lunchtime, it always begins using a dish known as Khar. Khar also identifies the primary ingredient in the dish, which can be an alkali extracted from the banana peels of the variety referred to as Bhim Kol. The peels are dried out, roasted, and maintained, and before planning the dish, they are soaked in tepid to warm water to secure a brownish filtrate, which is usually then found in cooking food. The dish could be made out of different ingredients; however, the one made out of natural papaya is definitely most cherished, referred to as Amitar Khar. If uncooked papaya isn't obtainable after that, cabbage or squash can be used as well. Occasionally, a fried seafood head can be scrambled into the dish through the later on stages from the food preparation process. Khar is certainly thought to be best for the belly, easing digestion.

If you have been indulging in excessive reddish meats and processed foods, isn't it about time you included some alkaline food in what you eat? Here is a list to truly get you started.

Green Leafy Vegetables

The majority of green leafy vegetables are thought to come with an alkaline effect inside our system. It isn't without reason our elders and wellness experts always recommend us to add greens inside our daily food diet. They contain important minerals that are essential for your body to handle various processes.

Cauliflower and Broccoli

If you value sautéed broccoli in Asian spices or gobi matar, they may be both healthy. They contain a number of phytochemicals that are crucial for the body. Toss it up with various other vegetables like capsicum, coffee beans, and green peas, and you possess your health dosage right there.

Citrus Fruits

Contrary to the fact that citric fruits are highly acidic and could have an acidic influence on your body, they will be the best way to obtain alkaline foods. Lemon, lime, and oranges contain Vitamin C, and so they are recognized to assist in detoxifying the machine, including providing rest from acidity.

Seaweed and Ocean Salt

Did you know seaweed or ocean vegetables have 10-12 times more mineral content material than those grown on land? Also, they are regarded as highly alkaline meal sources, and so are known to produce various advantages to the body program. You can suggest adding nori or kelp to the plate of soup, or make sushi at home. Or simply sprinkle some ocean salt into the salads, soups, omelets, etc.

Root Vegetables

Underlying vegetables like fairly sweet potato, beets, and carrots are excellent resources of alkali. They taste greatest when roasted with just a little sprinkling of spices and additional seasonings. Frequently, these are overcooked, making them miss out almost all their goodness. Give consideration while cooking, and you'll fall deeply in love with root vegetables as you figure out how to use them in soups, stir-fries, salads, and more.

Seasonal Fruits

Every nutritionist and wellness expert will let you know that adding seasonal fruits in your diet can be beneficial to your wellbeing. They come filled with nutritional vitamins, nutrients, and antioxidants that look after various functions in the stomach. They may be good alkaline meal sources too.

Nuts

Don't you love to chew on nut products when food cravings activate? Besides being resources of great fats, in addition, they create an alkaline impact in the stomach. However, being that they are high in calorie consumption, it's important to have limited levels of nut products. Add cashews, chestnuts, and almonds inside your daily meal strategy.

Onion, Garlic clove, and Ginger

Being among the most important ingredients in Indian cooking food, onion, garlic, and ginger are excellent flavor enhancers too. You should use them in various different ways – garlic clove to liven up your early morning toast, grated ginger within your soup or tea, newly sliced up onions in salads, etc.

CHAPTER 22: HERBAL HEALING

N‌ow you can begin your own regular routine of herbal healing, which means you know how to use the food you consume as medicine to treat the things that ail you, the chronic conditions that lead to chronic diseases, and keep you in overall poor health. Herbal medicine is also known as herbalism, and it is based on consuming parts of plants to heal you.

Drinking teas made from herbs is one of the best and easiest ways to use herbs and plants for health, besides eating food that is good for you. You can also use plants in other ways for your health. You can make an infusion of a part of a plant by steeping it in hot water for a period of time. When you add chopped bits of plants to cold water and allow it to stand and steep for longer time periods, this is known as maceration. When using this method, the water will absorb the minerals from the plant parts. When you boil the roots or the bark of the plant, you have made a decoction. Any of these methods can be used with any plant, and the liquid that comes from these methods will be full of minerals and vitamins that will keep you healthy.

You may already be using herbal preparations in your everyday life without knowing you are doing it. An extract is a preparation of herbs where tinctures are distilled into an extract. A tincture is made when you mix the herb with one hundred percent pure ethanol and allow it to be steep. The longer it steeps, the stronger the tincture will be. Completed tinctures have an alcohol content that will measure at least twenty-five percent. The percentage of alcohol in an extract is even less than the alcohol content of a tincture. So if you have ever cooked a dish that calls for using pure vanilla extract, pure lemon extract, pure maple extract, etc., you have used an herbal preparation.

And while Americans are becoming better at using herbal medicines on a daily basis, the Asians and Europeans have centuries of practice to draw on. These are the things that Dr. Sebi tried to teach his followers. The art of being healthy goes beyond just eating healthy foods, although that is an important part of the equation. It is important that everything you do for yourself will help to keep you healthy. People from China and India are particularly good at compounding herbs, a process which refers to mixing several herbs in a particularly balanced formula in order to provide treatment for a specific problem. These are formulas that have been used for thousands of years and are quite effective in their treatment of ailments. But the goal of using these compounds is not just to treat a specific disease or relieve a specific symptom. The goal of botanical medicine is to create changes in your body that are designed to make your body chemistry work better and to be in better balance so that a permanent cure and a healthier life can be achieved and maintained. And the particular compound used is generally tailored to the particular needs of that individual, so there is no one formula that is prescribed to all. This is one of the goals of the Alkaline Diet, to teach you how to mix different foods together to suit your particular needs.

Herbal medicine, or herbalism as it is frequently referred to, consists of using the roots, berries, flowers, bark, leaves, and seeds of the plants to create a product that is used for medicinal purposes. These concepts go along with the concepts of the Alkaline Diet. While the use of herbal medicine fell out of favor in some industrialized countries in recent years, it is beginning to come back into favor. With the rise of the Alkaline Diet and the teachings of Dr. Sebi, the world is beginning to see the sense behind the use of plants and plant-based products to keep themselves healthy, the way traditional medicine has taught for centuries.

You will find many benefits to using herbal medicines besides the medicines themselves. Herbs will rarely have harmful side effects when they are used in the proper dosage, while many prescription medicines have adverse side effects that are often worse than the condition that they are trying to treat. Medicines that are made from herbs will use the natural healing process of your own body to treat chronic conditions. The herbs you will be using are simple ingredients that are already made by your body. And herbal medicine is quite inexpensive, whereas modern medicine can be very expensive. Herbs are generally available almost anywhere. Some of the more simple herbs can be grown at home as people do in less industrialized parts of the world. You might not always know when you have already used a topical form of herbal medicine, but if you have ever used a lotion with aloe vera gel as one of the ingredients, then you have used an herbal remedy. Things that you might use every day will have medicinal properties.

- Ginseng is taken as a tea to relieve respiratory and digestive issues.

- Anise seed is made into a tea to relieve chest congestion.

- Basil eaten with food will help to settle a digestive upset and will help to improve a sluggish appetite.

- Black pepper will stimulate your taste buds, stimulate your digestive systems so it will perform more efficiently, and will help to clear out congestions of the lungs and sinuses.

- Cayenne pepper will stimulate your basic metabolic rate and help reduce bad cholesterol in your blood.

- Chamomile is gentle enough to use daily. As a tea, it will help you sleep, and when added to your bath, it will help you relax, and it will also help to soothe tired muscles.

- Cinnamon will help to relieve heartburn and bloating, and it might help to reduce your blood sugar levels.

- Coconut oil helps to increase your energy levels and to balance your hormones.

- Cranberry makes a delicious tea that will help to prevent tooth decay and relieve problems in your urinary tract.

- Echinacea tea will help prevent or treat infections of your throat or mouth and will also help relieve the symptoms of colds and sinus congestions.

- Eucalyptus tea will help to clear out congested lungs and sinuses, and it can also help to relieve the pain and stiffness that is associated with arthritis.

- Olive oil will reduce the risk to develop cardiovascular disease.

- Peppermint is a delicious herb that will help relieve gas and bloating, chronic indigestion, headaches, and muscle aches.

- Pumpkin seeds have compounds that will help to heal skin irritations.

- Rosemary can be used to season your food or made into tea. Either way, it will help relieve arthritis pain and muscle aches.

- Sage used in your recipes will help with your digestive issues, and if you make it into tea, it will help relieve fevers and symptoms of the common cold.

- Sesame will help your body to have lower blood pressure and lower bad cholesterol.

- Thyme will make your food taste great while helping calm your coughing or easing your lung congestion.

- Turmeric has long been known to relieve inflammation.

You can easily add more herbs into your daily diet so that the foods that you eat will help heal your body while making your food taste wonderful. Every time that you go to the grocery store, you should check out one or two new herbs that you have not tried before. When you make it a habit to buy herbs on a regular basis, then you will be creating the habit of using them in your recipes on a regular basis. You might even want to try your hand at growing an herb garden, even if it is just a few pots of herbs sitting in the window of your kitchen. Even someone who lives in an apartment can find space to grow a few herbs. And if the fresh herbs are right there where you are cooking, then you will be more likely to use them regularly. Fresh herbs will have more of the compounds that will make your food taste good while they heal your body.

If you buy your herbs in bulk, you may find that you will save time and money in preparing them. When you buy the herbs, plan to prepare them all at the same time. If you are trying to chop the herb and it won't easily chop, then it might not be dry enough. It is an easy matter to save leftover herbs and extra herbs. One excellent way to store herbs is to freeze them into ice cubes. This method will serve two purposes. It will give you a way to safely store the herb, and it will give you frozen herbs in ice cubes to add to your morning smoothies.

Herbs help promote a relaxing environment, so your body will give support to your mental, emotional, and physical rejuvenation and stability. Herbs will set the foundation to heal illnesses and diseases, and to help to prevent chronic diseases from ever developing. Herbs can be used in many different combinations to give assistance to the same area of the body or to fight the same condition. Herbs can assist with the health of a wide array of conditions and can be beneficial to several organs all at once. This is good because no organ in your body works by itself, but all of your organs and systems are interconnected in some way. When you combine herbs to set a target at a specific illness or a particular area of the body, it will increase the overall effectiveness of the herb in its ability to heal your body. Herbs are an important part of the Alkaline Diet.

CHAPTER 23: TIPS AND TRICKS

Be Mentally and Psychologically Ready

Eating food is a daily routine that human beings are supposed to undergo. The nature of substances and foods that we consume every day can result in a lifetime consumption habit if it is not regulated. Once the habits form, it is difficult to disband them. People surrounding us can also influence your habits or hinder transformation. So before jumping into the alkaline lifestyle, you need to think more about it. It will help you avoid making empty promises to yourself. After you have already thought about moving to the alkaline diet, look into the obstacles that will prevent you either psychologically or mentally in your transformation journey. With the knowledge in the distractions, chances of successfully getting inducted to the diet are high.

Drink More Water

Consumption of water into the body is vital. Water helps in maintaining brain health and other body operations. There are herbs in Dr. Sebi's diet that contain laxative effects that boost the removal of toxic substances through the urine. So, you need to replace the water that is used in the process. You should always be hydrated. The doctor here recommends taking in spring water since they are normally in an alkaline state. Tap water is often contaminated with chemicals such as chloride compounds and other chemicals.

According to the doctor, one should drink a gallon of spring water on the minimum daily. Avoid taking water containing softeners. Water from reverse osmosis systems should be avoided too. The work of the water is to help in nutrient absorption and organ and joint cushioning. Remember that existing health organizations do recommend the intake of a gallon of water as well.

You should also make drinking water a habit.

Include Extra Whole Meals to Your Diet

The whole foods range from the fruits that you like to fresh fish fillets. You should distance yourself from consuming foods that are kept in packages as they are very addictive. Restraining from these foods will greatly assist you as you advance through the alkaline diet.

Work very hard in completely substituting the processed meals with the whole foods. A lot of processed foods contain sugars that are enhanced. The sugars are considered very addictive as they can trigger cravings for the foods.

Read The Ingredient Labels

Avoiding other types of foods can be difficult most times. So, you can resort to reading the labels of the products to know the ingredients in them. It keeps you in the know-how of what you take into your body. The habit also assists in directing you in what to change from the foods you eat. It will also assist you once you have fully embraced Dr. Sebi's diet. Here, you will be in the know of whatever you consumed.

Pay Attention To The Snacks

You should avoid taking packed snacks from the store.

Since you are not supposed to take packed snacks from the stores, it does not mean that you should stop consuming snacks. You just need to take snacks in the right way. You can try preparing some on your own. The snacks can be a mixture of raisins, walnuts, or other fruits that have been dried.

Review The Approved Foods

Look into the non-recommended foods in the diet. Avoid them in every possible way that you can. When you are prepared mentally for the recommended foods, you will easily get used to them.

CONCLUSION

D r. Sebi's diet method involved using herbs and natural alkaline plant-based foods to alkalize the body. This helps return the body again to a state of homeostasis.

The diet was made up of only natural alkaline vegetables, nuts, fruits, alkaline grains, and legumes, which could alkalize and get rid of mucus from the body. Besides the diet, he also made use of natural alkaline herbs to detoxify the body's cells on the intracellular and intercellular level.

This alkaline diet is totally based on the idea that sickness can most effectively exist in an acidic environment. The body works to keep a marginally alkaline 7.4 pH environment in the blood.

Blood is the point of equilibrium for homeostasis, but if the body becomes too acidic, it will use alkaline minerals and compounds from bones and fluids from the body to keep the blood's pH level stable. This endangers the health of various parts of the body and results in the development of new sicknesses and diseases.

Many people claim that the way we live and our culture today are incredibly harmful to our wellbeing. They conclude that consuming highly acidic products affects the quality of cells and body fluids. Sadly, this evidence was not applied in several clinical studies, although there were a variety of individuals who attempted alkaline diets and recorded impressive health benefits.

Alkaline diets and plant-based diets of Dr. Sebi can give some of theise health benefits: increased vitality, weight control, lower dependency or no insulin reliance on patients with diabetes, no acid reflux, enhancement in hair, nails, eyes, better sleeping habits, mental stability, candida symptoms relief and just to name a couple.

This regime decreases body contaminants and inspires general well-being. It will help you take a harmless, healthier approach to food. It will also reduce the chances of other diseases. If you have to lose weight, it can motivate you to do it easily and reliably. This is related to improve the strength and resilience that everyone requires.

The food and herbs listed are just a few of the herbs Dr. Sebi makes use of in his products.

Dr. Sebi doesn't support the use of the word protein. He took this position primarily to counteract the industry's manipulation that has made many people think protein is the most important nutrient to consume. He made a strong point that iron in plants is the most important nutrient because the health of the blood is built on iron. The blood supplies oxygen and nutrients to support all metabolic functions.

Researchers found out that Dr. Sebi's method and the herbs that he used have been a part of alkaline food lists that went round the internet world, and that had been utilized by many herbal practitioners.

Traditional healing herbs used by Dr. Sebi include dandelion, sarsaparilla, and burdock root, which cleanse the blood and the liver. The world-famous and growing holistic health movements now extensively use these herbs.

Dr. Sebi's diet is an entirely new approach to food. As such, it might be hard to get used to it, especially at the start.

It is advisable to try Dr. Sebi's method for at least 30 days if you do not fully adopt a new dietary regime. Engage for a month and see the improvements.

After a month, you might want to switch to this diet entirely!

Printed in Great Britain
by Amazon

56380797R00084